Atif Zafar is a neurologist, a researcher, an entrepreneur, an advocate, mentor, coach, and a life-long student of science and leadership. In this book, he shares his insights and perspective on physician leadership and why the evolution of physician-mindset in the current healthcare system is crucial. In this book, he wishes to converse with medical students, trainees, early career physicians, and other stake holders to stimulate a transformative discussion and to instigate leadership. These discussions aim to introduce the core principles of leadership for the future generations of doctors, and to foment a culture of leadership in this incisive, analytical, bright and smart faction of the society.

Contributing authors: Dr. Mudassir Farooqui, M.P.H. and Dr. Syed A. Quadri.

Content Contribution & Improvement: Theresa Simpson.

Proof reading and Editorial expertise by Lyndsay Wilson.

PURPLEYE PRESS 2020

Copyright 2019 Atif Zafar. All rights reserved.

No part of this book may be reproduced in any form or by any electronic or mechanical means, including information storage and retrieval systems, without permission in writing from the publisher. The only exception is by a reviewer, who may quote short excerpts in a published review.

ISBN PAPERBACK: 978-1-7341676-2-7

Library of Congress Control Number: 2019916439

Cover Design by Purpleye Press

Interior Organization by Purpleye Press

Printed in the USA.

The information presented herein represents the view of the author as of the date of publication. This book is presented for information purposes only. Due to the rate at which conditions change, the author reserves the right to alter and update his opinions based on new conditions. While every attempt has been made to verify the information in this book, neither the author nor his affiliates/partners assume any responsibility for errors, inaccuracies, or omissions.

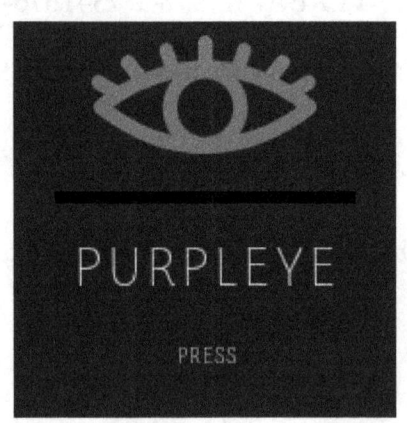

TO THE FOUR EXCEPTIONAL WOMEN WHO INSPIRE ME EVERY DAY:

MY MOTHER, MY WIFE, MY DAUGHTER, & MY SISTER!

CONTENTS

INTRODUCTION 12

BACKGROUND ON PHYSICIANS AS ADVOCATES 19

BACKGROUND ON PHYSICIANS AS RESEARCHERS 20

BACKGROUND ON PHYSICIANS AS ADMINISTRATORS 21

BACKGROUND ON PHYSICIANS AS ENTREPRENEURS 22

BACKGROUND ON PHYSICIANS AS QUALITY IMPROVEMENT LEADERS 23

PHYSICIANS AS ADVOCATES AND POLICYMAKERS 24

ADVOCACY - WHAT DOES IT MEAN? 24

IS PHYSICIAN ADVOCACY IMPORTANT? 28

SUN PROTECTION 30

BARRIERS TO PHYSICIANS ADVOCACY 31

ADVOCACY AS PART OF THE MEDICAL

CURRICULUM   32

IMPRESSIVE WAYS PHYSICIANS CAN TAKE CONTROL AS POLICY MAKERS   35

PHYSICIANS AS RESEARCHERS   39

HOW TO DEVELOP INTEREST IN RESEARCH   39

IDENTIFY AN AREA OF INTEREST OR SOMETHING THAT PERSONALLY AFFECTS YOU   40

IDENTIFY AND JOIN ACTIVE RESEARCH NETWORKS   41

GET A RESEARCH MENTOR   41

EXPLORE NEW (AND MORE!) PROBLEMS   42

WHY ALL PHYSICIANS SHOULD BE RESEARCHERS   44

THE IMPACT OF RESEARCH ON PHYSICIANS   48

BENEFITS AND DOWNSIDES OF DOING RESEARCH – PERSONAL AND PROFESSIONAL LEVEL 53

THE BENEFITS 53

THE DOWNSIDES 54

HOW TO JUGGLE THE RESEARCH AND CLINICAL ASPECTS OF A PHYSICIAN'S WORKING LIFE 56

EFFECTIVE TIME MANAGEMENT AND ORGANIZATIONAL SKILLS 57

EFFECTIVE PROFESSIONAL COMMUNICATION 57

MENTORSHIP 58

AVOIDING FEELINGS OF INFERIORITY IN EITHER ROLE 58

PHYSICIANS AS ADMINISTRATORS 59

CLINICAL AND ADMINISTRATIVE ROLES 61

THE RISE OF THE HOSPITAL ADMINISTRATOR 62

A CALL TO ACTION - WHAT PHYSICIANS MUST DO 64

PHYSICIANS AS ENTREPRENEURS 68

WHAT IS A PHYSICIAN

ENTREPRENEUR? 69

PHYSICIAN-ENTREPRENEURS AS ENTREPRENEURS 72

PHYSICIAN ENTREPRENEURS AS INTRAPRENEURS 73

TIPS FOR THE PHYSICIAN ENTREPRENEUR 74

WHY THE RISING NEED FOR PHYSICIAN-ENTREPRENEURS? 78

PHYSICIANS AS QUALITY IMPROVEMENT LEADERS 82

ESSENTIALS OF QUALITY IMPROVEMENT 82

PHYSICIANS AS MANAGERS 84

OVERVIEW 84

PROBLEMS WITH PHYSICIANS MANAGEMENT SKILLS 88

PHYSICIANS AS STRATEGIC MANAGERS 89

DEVELOPING ROBUST MANAGEMENT SKILLS AS A PHYSICIAN 93

POLICY AND POLITICAL PROCESSES 96

MANAGING AND DEVELOPING OTHERS 96

BALANCE OF PATIENT-FOCUSED AND PHYSICIAN-FRIENDLY APPROACHES 97

QUALITY IMPROVEMENT 97

PROGRAM DEFINITION AND MANAGEMENT 97

HOW TO ACQUIRE A STRATEGIC PERSPECTIVE 98

PHYSICIANS AS HR MANAGERS 100

THE IMPORTANCE OF HUMAN RESOURCES MANAGEMENT IN HEALTHCARE 101

PHYSICIANS AS LEADERS 104

PHYSICIAN LEADERSHIP SKILLS 104

ORGANIZATIONAL BEHAVIOR SKILLS 105

MOTIVATION 105

EFFECTIVE COMMUNICATION SKILLS 108

TEAM BUILDING 109

CONFLICT MANAGEMENT 111

CULTURE DEVELOPMENT 113

ANALYTICAL SKILLS 115

QUALITY CONTROL 116

RISK MANAGEMENT 117

FINANCIAL EXPERTISE 117

TRANSFORMING DOCTORS INTO LEADERS 120

WHEN THE LEADER ISN'T READY 122

WHEN THE LEADER HAS NO TIME TO PAUSE 123

THE DYAD MODEL 123

FUTURE PROSPECTS 127

CONCLUSION 130

CHAPTER 1

INTRODUCTION

A great number of physicians do not entirely comprehend the business of health care. Several times a week, an average physician cures disease, ameliorates health problems, fixes bones, carries out surgeries, and institutes a range of therapeutic and lifesaving interventions. We consider our jobs to be "saving lives," and we do our best in our everyday medical practice. However, considering present realities, merely saving lives within the confines of the hospital or clinic is not enough. Unfortunately, most physicians are content with their current limited roles in the healthcare system, choosing not to concern themselves with the bigger picture. It's a good thing to feel satisfied with our jobs, but not when the feeling of satisfaction comes at a great cost not just to the physician community but also to the patients we serve. We consciously limit our roles in healthcare to mere day-to-day medical practice which mostly involves pills, surgeries, and therapy. For the better part of our careers, we neglect policies, prices, and interaction with authorities as it relates to healthcare.

As doctors, people entrust us with their health. Many lives depend on our decisions. Consequently the decisions we make, and our willingness to make them, impacts the health and well-being of communities, and frankly the whole nation. We are entrusted with much more than the responsibilities of diagnosis and treatment. While it is easier to merely diagnose and treat disease and let the system take care of the rest, we cannot afford to continue with this ostrich mentality any longer. Our patients look to us to do what is in their "best interest," which is increasingly acquiring a new meaning. Our responsibilities toward our patients as well as to ourselves encompass a wide range of activities previously considered out of our scope of work. We owe it to our patients to be proactive in effecting change in ways that will have far-reaching impact on healthcare in general.

Just a few decades ago, smallpox, poliomyelitis, and leprosy ravaged towns, cities, and entire nations, taking the lives of innocent children and breadwinners alike. Fortunately, we now live in a world where those health problems have to a great extent been eliminated thanks to advances in prevention and treatment strategies such as accessible vaccines and cheaper medications. Furthermore, we have made technological advancements like air ambulances that can safely and rapidly transport sick and injured patients hundreds of miles away to well-equipped hospitals.

All of this is possible as a result of gradual progress in healthcare over the course of the last several centuries. While this kind of progress in healthcare continues, physicians are now obligated to begin making progress of a different kind, well beyond the confines of traditional medical practice. As physicians, we are one of, if not *the* most important players in healthcare. It then increasingly dawns on us to face our most important role in the society - which is providing good health care to populations - with a different perspective.

Since it is reasonably well-established that technological innovations, lower prices, improved healthcare delivery, and patient-focused research can help solve problems within healthcare systems and enhance provision of better medical care to patients, how then can physicians participate in this? How can they help lower drug prices for their patients? How can they help realize affordable healthcare? How can they help catalyze technological innovations in healthcare?

The questions are many, but one common answer lies within physician participation in leadership within healthcare systems. Physicians are uniquely positioned to lead healthcare organizations because they are committed to providing medical care to patients through treatment and prevention of diseases. A study by the London School of Economics found that healthcare institutions with the most physician involvement in management affairs performed considerably better. These institutions were more likely to experience improved effectiveness in general management, performance management, and general leadership as compared with hospitals with little physician leadership.

While there is traditionally a contentious and often conflicted relationship between hospital administrators and clinical practitioners, a leader with a clinical background (a physician leader) gives a healthcare institution credibility and introduces more trust among administrative and medical staff. A clinical background provides physician leaders with skills that allow them to respond to administrative problems in ways that are consistent with present clinical realities. A combination of leadership training with clinical expertise positions physician leaders as powerful and influential leaders capable of instigating relevant changes, seeing new possibilities, breaking down silos, inspiring others, and bringing to life dynamic healthcare visions for organizations.

It's true that some healthcare institutions and medical schools have recently made impressive efforts in providing coherent and relevant leadership training. However, what passes for leadership skills training in most hospitals and medical schools is a jumble of incomplete classes that lack any logical progression, coherence, and relevance. Sadly, the nature and organization of these lectures means they fail to truly develop market-ready, industry-relevant, and effective physician leaders.

This means that graduating physicians are not armed with the necessary skills and competencies needed to pilot the affairs of real-world departments or health care organizations. The average physician may lack the financial, motivational, risk management, communication, and team building skills needed to lead in the healthcare system. In medical school, we were all trained to be pediatricians, orthodontists, cardiovascular surgeons, optometrists, and so on. We were not trained to be managing partners, heads of department, chiefs of staff or medical directors within the field of healthcare. After all, all we wanted was to be doctors, not leaders.

This is why I wrote this book. To speak to all those brilliant medical students, residents, fellows, and early career physicians out there, and invite them to change their perspectives. Sometimes we find ourselves forced into the position of leadership; this unfortunately results in mediocre performance. The responsibilities and complexities of modern health care organizations are far too important to be left to "accidental leaders." The emergence of physician leaders in healthcare must therefore be deliberately cultivated. Leadership focused physician development programs must be accepted as a necessary part of a much larger, system-wide shift in healthcare. This will require a fundamental re-examination of our structures, priorities, and professional relationships in our current healthcare institutions. We must, for instance, rethink their governance structures and criteria for physician recruitment and promotion. Until that happens, the onus is on you.

The idea that doctors should function only as doctors is simply unfortunate and, on a personal level, rather disappointing. While it's true that some doctors in the U.S. have become senators, congress people, health secretaries and such, there's a dearth of physicians who could match the likes of Dr. Martin Luther King. I've undoubtedly been encouraged by prominent leaders in other parts of the world such as the inspiring Malaysian Dr. Mahathir Muhammed (a physician), the "founding father of the Chinese nation" Sun Yat-sen (a physician), national hero of the Philippines Jose Rizal (an ophthalmologist), three times Norwegian Prime Minister Gro Harlem Brundtland (a physician) and even the Argentinian Marxist revolutionary Che Guevara (also a physician). But the relative absence of such exemplary leadership from U.S. trained physicians is a question I have yet to find a satisfying answer for. Is it because we are forced to stay shackled to bureaucratic and legislative regulations, never getting the chance to think outside of the medical box? Or is it that we ourselves have come to expect so much less from the work we offer the world?

As modern physicians, we need to get smart and teach ourselves other non-medical skills. Whether it's management, sales, coding, marketing or administration, taking responsibility for innovative thinking and leadership is just part and parcel of our full role. Seminars, coaching events, online courses, networking with the right people – there are more avenues available to us than ever before. I believe now is the time for doctors to implement efficient, high-value and sustainable programs, and prepare themselves to lead the healthcare system into an accessible and affordable future for our patients.

A better trained physician workforce will help to rectify the current system. The relationship between physicians and health care organizations must be strengthened, the trust between them must be renewed, their visions reevaluated, and their mutual expectations must be clarified. And this ought to be initiated by physicians themselves. Manager-run institutions and their executives will automatically see physician leaders as equal and important partners in efficient healthcare delivery and overall organizational efficiency.

As the organizational structure transforms for the better, there must be increased attention towards identifying high-potential physicians and grooming them through formal development programs. And this will just be the beginning of how doctors can more proactively shape the future of healthcare, rather than passively being on the receiving end, along with the patients. There is a reason that insurance and pharmaceutical companies have taken control of our healthcare system, while the two most important entities, i.e. doctors and patients, are left frustrated and powerless at how things are developing.

With this book, I hope to offer insight into the different perspectives on physician leadership, into our changing involvement in enhancing healthcare, and into ways we can begin to take back control. It will provide the reader with a point of reference on what it actually means to become a leader in healthcare. I'll explore physician leadership through various paradigms, ranging from physicians as advocates, teachers, and entrepreneurs to fusion perspectives and how they can shape effective leaders in healthcare. I am hopeful my effort and passion for what doctors are truly capable of translates into a growing number of individuals feeling more aware, prepared, and motivated to transform the way we think and work. Eventually, impact on the lives of our patients is what I hope to accomplish. It's natural to think that as doctors become serious stakeholders in the healthcare system, patient experiences and outcome would drastically improve.

Below is a succinct preview on the structure of this text and information covered.

BACKGROUND ON PHYSICIANS AS ADVOCATES

Rather than just being good medical experts, we must position ourselves as advocates for improvement within healthcare systems. I have been inspired by advances in medical care that go beyond the confines of traditional practice; to keep pace with this, we must also be willing to go beyond traditional medical practice. To be advocates for improvement, we must seek to find ways to solve problems beyond using pills, syringes or surgical knives. Air ambulances are a prime example of the scope of our responsibilities in healthcare. While they've saved many lives, they've also driven many patients to bankruptcy. Regulations on air ambulances are quite lax, meaning operators can charge patients enormous amounts of money. This is quite profitable for those involved, but devastating for financially disadvantaged patients.

I remember a 64-year-old patient who, while recovering from a hemorrhagic stroke, began suffering from excruciating pain in his right hemibody, i.e. the rare phenomenon called post-stroke pain syndrome. I prescribed him Lyrica, an expensive medication which his insurance approved, but only for a 60-day supply, no refills. His pain improved, and he continue with aggressive outpatient therapy. But of course, when his Lyrica eventually ran out, he returned to the clinic to discuss cheaper alternatives. I remember spending months trying out other medications like amitriptyline, gabapentin, and venlafaxine, but nothing else worked. Eventually, after his insurance company's repeated refusal to cover Lyrica, he was started on Botox injections to help with the spasticity. Thankfully, the pain slowly became more tolerable. As a physician, I had "solved" my patient's problem. However, the real impediment was far bigger than simply selecting the right medication. I found myself questioning the health of the entire system, and my obligations to my patients to work to improve that system.

As physicians, our responsibility is to our patients' health and general wellbeing within the system. Doesn't the onus then fall on us to make air ambulances cheaper for all? Isn't it our business to make sure that our patients have realistic access to medications that will drastically improve their quality of life? This is what I mean by advocacy, and as physicians, I believe it's crucial that we all become advocates.

BACKGROUND ON PHYSICIANS AS RESEARCHERS

Research is the backbone of science and technology. As physicians genuinely strive to improve healthcare, they can use their medical expertise to participate, influence or steer research towards more patient-focused solutions. Since physicians usually know what matters practically on the frontlines, their experience should be appreciated and used in research to identify "relevant details" and provide "valuable insights" on what should and should not be done. We can also analyze the validity of the decades-old belief that medical research should be separated from medical practice, and that physicians should avoid "mixing up" the two disciplines.

BACKGROUND ON PHYSICIANS AS ADMINISTRATORS

An issue which initially piqued my interest in physician leadership (or the sad lack thereof) was what I observed to be a kind of "crisis of office space." In my department, I saw non-physician administrative leadership in separate office spaces, while most of the senior faculty (my mentors included) were made to share office space with colleagues, the reasoning being that the hospital was short on space. Despite physicians being the main revenue generators of the hospital, and indeed supporting the salaries of the administrative staff, the very building layout did not reflect this. I could only wonder if this organizational discrepancy spoke to a deeper issue concerning physicians and the space allotted to their leadership.

When I share this sentiment with colleagues, most agree that providing physicians with office space never used to be a problem, but that recently accommodations have been made to increasing demands from administration. Pursuing grants, searching for specialized expertise, and courting academic prestige are obviously prioritized, with the physicians playing the role of workhorses only, doing as they're told, sitting where they're told to sit, and writing notes as they're regulated to. Though it's an uncharitable assessment, my growing feeling in observing all this was that doctors' immense skills were going to waste as they were manipulated as mere pawns by those for whom the bottom line is all that counts.

As physicians, we try our best to beat the odds and provide the best medical care we can, but at some point, our efforts as mere physicians is not enough. Sometimes, we find that we possess the desire to improve our immediate organizations (hospitals or healthcare centers) in ways that would positively impact the health of the immediate population. This brings up the need to not just influence but actively participate in steering organizational policies towards more patient-oriented approaches.

There is a great need for medical expertise in making decisions or policies on which healthcare systems are run. Clearly, this requires physicians' participation in the administration of healthcare organizations.

BACKGROUND ON PHYSICIANS AS ENTREPRENEURS

In today's world, entrepreneurship is becoming more important in healthcare than ever before. Rising drug costs, competing needs, and several system-wide inefficiencies in healthcare means that even the government and established healthcare institutions cannot do everything that's needed to improve healthcare. More than ever, it has become increasingly important for physicians, armed with their wealth of practical experience and academic knowledge, to independently participate in creating solutions and innovations in healthcare to solve these inefficiencies.

Physician entrepreneurship opens up a world of opportunity for technological innovation and "new ways of doing things" with the ultimate goal of improving healthcare. Physicians' participation in the business frontier of healthcare is essential. It's irrelevant whether their participation is influenced by the need for additional streams of income or solely for creating positive impact, as long as there's improved efficiency within the system and improvement in the all-important health outcomes.

BACKGROUND ON PHYSICIANS AS QUALITY IMPROVEMENT LEADERS

Quality improvement is necessary for optimizing healthcare delivery and ultimately, patient satisfaction. It's essential that physicians assume an active role in quality improvement within healthcare organizations. It's important for physician leaders to identify solutions and make conscious efforts to improve on these solutions. As physicians, we are part of a system that is experiencing rising drug costs and a greater need for patient-focused efficiency. It's important for physicians to step in as quality improvement leaders to genuinely improve "solutions" in the quest for a better healthcare system. We must strive for improvement in quality of medical services, in performance both in medical practice and in leadership, and find ways to provide better healthcare at affordable rates. Quality improvement realistically means shorter length of stay for patients, minimal readmission rates, minimal errors in diagnosis, low recurrence or relapse of disease, and improved physician-patient relationships.

CHAPTER 2

PHYSICIANS AS ADVOCATES AND POLICYMAKERS

In this book, our ultimate goal is to prepare your mind as a physician for leadership roles. Advocacy is undeniably an important aspect of leadership. As physicians, we are introduced to advocacy quite early in our careers; first by the idea subtly trickling in, but we all eventually catch up. Understanding what advocacy entails in our everyday practice is important to achieve competency in our jobs as healthcare professionals. It's important to approach our jobs in the healthcare sector with the mind of an advocate, working for improvement that benefits not just us as physicians, but our patients and in fact all humankind. Physicians do not only have to advocate for patients, they also ought to advocate for *themselves*. They should advocate within their organization or practice for better salaries, better support services, modern tools, and improved infrastructures. It's vital to advocate through policymakers to influence policy changes at the state, national or even global level.

ADVOCACY - WHAT DOES IT MEAN?

Advocacy is the ability to identify the needs of an individual, group of individuals or a cause and then take informed decisions to support those needs.

As physicians we are privy to an honest and sometimes intimate knowledge of our patient's needs. Physicians are always on the front line and experience firsthand how system inadequacies impact the lives of our patients. We are uniquely positioned to understand what patients really need - well beyond the drugs, the therapy, and the special care. It then weighs heavily on us to use this knowledge to properly influence government policies and healthcare delivery mechanisms, and push past social barriers to ameliorate the problems of our patients. It's extremely important to us as physicians to learn to see a patient's need beyond a biomedical model and become accustomed to integrating social factors into healthcare delivery.

While advocacy could mean a lot of things to different people, to physicians, advocacy is simply positive influence – it's using the important knowledge we are trusted with or privileged to access to analyze the status quo and push for improvement. It's our conscious efforts to use this knowledge for stimulating social, economic and political change to neutralize threats to human health and general wellbeing.

Advocacy is a physician's social responsibility. The precursor to this is usually establishing a healthy patient-physician relationship to enable the physician to adequately understand the needs and priorities of the patient. It involves being present in the system to understand what is not right. As physicians, we must never assume that we fully understand a disadvantaged patient's need or priorities. We must instead strive always to be respectful and observant.

This does not mean intrusive or invasive, just subtly acquiring the information we would need. More often than not, this information is right there, staring at us; it just needs a little effort to notice. The most important thing is that we recognize this information and leverage it to create positive influence.

The breadth of advocacy is enormous and the frontiers to advocate are numerous. We can advocate for an individual patient, a group of patients or an entire community. We can advocate through creating awareness, through educational programs or by directly influencing policies. The channels and ways to advocate are truly numerous. For instance, individual patient advocacy may be targeted at their immediate medical or social health needs. This could include advocacy for housing, feeding, and social supports as well as providing referrals for addiction programs. Advocacy for a group of patients in an organizational setting may involve positively influencing the status quo or directly addressing organizational inadequacies. This may include pushing for improvement in quality of service, use of better tools, or formulation of favorable organization-level policies wherein change is affected to impact the health and wellbeing of a population. A more wide-reaching advocacy with greater impact is a community-, national- or system-level advocacy that aims to bring change to policies wherein an even greater population of patients and non-patients are affected. This kind of advocacy requires more than just helping individual patients get the medical or social services they need; it requires prudently working to address the root causes of the challenges they face.

Each physician's obligation to advocacy is usually grounded in their professional experience, area of expertise, and their duty to their patients. Just because physicians should be advocates, it doesn't mean they should advocate for *anything*. Even in the medical field, "physicians as advocates" does not necessarily entail a sector-wide advocacy. For instance, it won't be particularly reasonable to expect an ophthalmologist to advocate for child oral health, nor a dentist for better access to anti-retroviral medications. Though doing so would not entirely be a problem, advocacy is best realized in a familiar terrain where the physician has a semblance of expertise.

Physicians are generally trained and conditioned to be objective and apolitical. Furthermore, the values of scientific objectivity are quite pronounced in the medical field, which means physicians are sometimes hesitant to join the sphere of advocacy. It's certainly easy for us as physicians to convince ourselves that advocacy belongs to the world of politics, and that we should be concerned more about the immediate needs of our individual patients. Physicians can also argue that civic virtues and social responsibilities are outside the professional realm of being a physician. There are certainly real risks, which may include accusations of dabbling into politics, not maintaining neutrality, and the potential for employer retaliation. Furthermore, the work of a physician is exhausting and intense enough already; taking on an advocacy role in addition to being a good physician to your own patients can be daunting and time consuming.

However, taking on a task with a potential to impact change on a larger scale can be fulfilling and life changing. For many physicians, the words of Rudolf Virchow, the father of modern pathology, remain immortal: "Medicine is a social science, and politics is nothing else but medicine on a large scale. Medicine, as a social science, as the science of human beings, has the obligation to point out problems and to attempt their theoretical solution: the politician, the practical anthropologist, must find the means for their actual solution. The physicians are the natural attorneys of the poor, and social problems fall to a large extent within their jurisdiction."

IS PHYSICIAN ADVOCACY IMPORTANT?

The abysmal number of young and upcoming physicians who actively recognize the need to be advocates does not in any way undermine the importance of advocacy. Advocacy in healthcare seeks to ensure that people, particularly patients and those who are most vulnerable in society, are able to have their voices heard on issues that are critical and important to them. It seeks to ensure that they are defended, and their rights safeguarded. It's important that their views and wishes are honestly considered when decisions and policies that may directly or indirectly impact their lives are being made.

Generally, the first step to solving a problem is identifying the problem. For problems in healthcare, this involves recognizing that the problems even exist in the first place. Advocacy in healthcare creates widespread visibility for a problem. It alerts people to the existence of public health issues or creates awareness for researchers with potential to solve the problem. The more visibility a topic receives, the more likely it is to be a concern to the public and relevant authorities. Advocacy then effectively becomes a vehicle to gain access to politicians, legislators, health leaders, and corporate executives with the power and the means to effect positive change.

If we genuinely recognize the fact that physical, economic and social policies determine peoples' access to better healthcare, and that these policies are molded by decisions made by individuals, organizations, and governments, then it becomes quite important that physicians be engaged in making these decisions. It's extremely important that physicians play an active role either directly, as participants in the decision-making process, or indirectly, by creating awareness, providing information, and building constituencies to support a favorable course of action. When awareness is created within a community, much of the requirement to fix a problem is met. The likelihood of positive action being taken by relevant authorities to address a public health problem is significantly greater when self-aware and informed communities speak for themselves about problems and possible solutions.

To serve as a point of reference, it's possible to clearly identify examples of the effectiveness of advocacy in healthcare. Below is a highlighted example of this effectiveness. Effectiveness in this case is measured by success in changes to local or national laws, modification of organization level policies, and a general awareness of a problem.

SUN PROTECTION

In the early 1980s, evidence of the relationship between high rates of skin cancer and sun exposure at a young age was established by healthcare professionals. These healthcare professionals then started rigorous advocacy programs to create awareness of the problem and attempt to influence individuals and decision makers to adopt suggested solutions. Using their knowledge and wealth of experience on the problem, they developed mass media advertising campaigns which ran from 1985-1995. Over time, individuals voluntarily opted to protect themselves from the sun. As the awareness of the problem grew, the issue became a major public discussion, subsequently triggering gradual changes in policies across a range of sectors - notably education - where schools were obliged to provide more sun protection for their students. It also permeated industry practices with increased demand for protective clothing, increased sun protection factor in sunscreens, significantly reduced taxation on sunscreen products, and much more. All these results were made possible by advocacy carried out by a group of physicians which later resonated among parents, politicians, unions, and many other entities.

This is a classic example that demonstrates the effectiveness of advocacy through creating awareness and instigating community participation and engagement. This resulted in significant changes in government policies and people's attitude towards sun protection. So, it's safe to say that considering our current healthcare culture and realities of how modern societies work, it's not just important but essential that physicians actively participate in advocacy.

BARRIERS TO PHYSICIANS ADVOCACY

Despite the recognition, to some of extent, of the importance of a physician's participation in the political conversation, knowing how to put advocacy into practice remains rather problematic partly because it is undefined in scope and concept. Barriers to physicians' advocacy exist, and there are thoughtful perspectives on what these barriers could be. Some of them include the following:

One of the greatest barriers to physician's advocacy is that it's not considered as a professional imperative. Just as politicians take on the spirit of advocacy and consider it core to their professional responsibilities, so should physicians. If advocacy is to be a professional imperative, then it should definitely be treated as such in all spheres. Medical schools and graduate education programs for instance do not deliberately train physicians as advocates. Similarly, accrediting bodies do not clearly define advocacy competencies, and as such most systematically trained physicians do not possess even basic skills in advocacy. Even with widespread calls for physician advocacy, both undergraduate and graduate medical education institutions do little to nothing towards institutionalizing it.

Physicians tend to be considerably apolitical and are statistically less likely to be involved in politics and civil matters than other professions. There's a popular opinion that medical training largely isolates physicians from the community and indeed the general public during their (in)famously tedious and academically demanding training period. The inability of physicians to mentally delineate mainstream politics from advocacy in healthcare also presents a barrier to their willingness to participate. Healthcare is quite a demanding field and requires enormous time investment. Physicians are bombarded with daily demands. They may sometimes have the passion and zeal to transform care models and cultivate value-based, patient-driven systems, but unfortunately, they also feel plenty of pressure to improve revenue and cash flow. It then becomes quite difficult for practicing physicians to take on any responsibilities beyond the pressing health problem at hand. Finally, for would-be advocates, there is the unspoken fear of being ostracized and straying from the usual guidelines of evidence-based medical practice. This hugely impacts the willingness of physicians to be strong advocates.

ADVOCACY AS PART OF THE MEDICAL CURRICULUM

The system that exists today might not be fixed tomorrow, but taking essential steps to close the loopholes now will help willing physicians better foster advocacy skills. Advocacy was traditionally a trait observed in our predecessor physicians. New physicians began to observe its impacts and to develop similar behaviors as independent practitioners. Thus, physician advocacy gradually but steadily grew in strength. The importance of practicing physician advocates has perhaps been unappreciated to date, at least given their involvement in formal medical curricula. This is why it's important to integrate role model figures either directly or indirectly into medical practice as inspiration for younger physicians. Both trainees and established physician advocates must establish a healthy relationship to keep the flames of advocacy alive. The ability to productively liaise for improvements must be encouraged during the formative period of young physicians.

However, as counterintuitive as it might seem, the greatest way to foster physician advocacy skills remains advocacy itself, period. Let's consider a practical example of how advocacy for medical students could not only benefit the students themselves, but model for them an attitude of bigger-picture thinking that could carry over to their work as future physicians. One of the issues in academic hospitals is the lack of interest among graduating medical students towards neurology. Just out of curiosity, I interviewed a few dozen students to find out why. One reason was the lack of clinicians' involvement in the pre-clinical years, where typically PhDs drive the neuroscience sessions, meaning this topic inevitably becomes the most difficult for students. Another given reason was the lack of experience during the clerkship, and the overall ownership given to them for patient care by the neurologists.

Interviewing students for the reasons behind their lack of interest was certainly a good first step, but what was needed was a more thorough understanding of the issues behind these reasons, so they could be resolved. This could entail simplifying clinical neurology on bedsides, or having the department chair working with faculty to ensure there are actual clinicians presenting neurosciences to preclinical students in dynamic, engaging ways. If the entire department envisions attracting more students into neurology, these small changes in attitudes and priorities could do just that. Indirectly, students trained in such an environment will internalize the spirit of big-picture thinking and carry that sense of advocacy into their future careers. But a department that is overworked, and short on manpower and proper strategy can't offer this to its students, and, indirectly, to all the patients who will eventually depend on them.

Advocacy need not be a formal part of the curriculum to positively impact medical students' training. Rather, a system-wide approach during residency training can begin to impart on students the importance of thinking beyond their purely medical training. One of the challenges for interns and residents is surviving overnight call while maintaining collegiality with nurses, techs, and especially Emergency Medicine colleagues. Those who are unsuccessful often see an email sent by nursing staff to the program director regarding the resident's slow, terse, or downright rude response to pages. While most physicians are decent and caring human beings, the stress and lack of sleep that comes with an overnight call can often make them forget they are part of a larger team with a common goal: patient care. The idea is that while you manage a critical patient in ED, it's part of your job as a physician to ensure that all collaborators are "managed" professionally as part of a team. Just updating them by saying, "I'm managing a critical patient down in ER, and would appreciate if you could hold the fort for a little bit" would help. If you have a patient crashing to the floor, asking a senior nurse to call the rapid response team will ensure the safety of the patient while helping everyone keep their cool. These "skills" don't appear in the curriculum, yet go a long way to engaging the system beyond merely being a physician and working directly with colleagues towards the goal that matters most: patient wellbeing.

If more medical institutions are to take advocacy seriously, then existing physicians' advocates must push passionately for such. If relevant educational institutions are to include advocacy in their curriculum, then existing physicians must advocate for such. Much more awareness of the subject matter must be created to the "physician public." Much more pressure must be thrust against relevant authorities. It will then inevitably become a (political) liability for them if they refuse to act.

IMPRESSIVE WAYS PHYSICIANS CAN TAKE CONTROL AS POLICY MAKERS

The decisions made and policies formulated within a medical community or organization resonates across the larger community. For example, a surgeon's choice to use a particular technique for a certain operation are conditioned by prior decisions, such as the number and types of operating rooms available for use, types of equipment available in the organization, the quality and expertise of hired surgical assistants, and a range of other policy influenced actions. The surgeon's decision may also be influenced by prior decisions made by the hospital's quality assurance committee. To put it succinctly, decisions involving individual clinical judgment during administration of healthcare and decisions involving larger organization-wide policy issues are highly interrelated. This further collaborates the notion that the line between "clinical' and " administrative" decision making is dangerously thin. It then becomes important for physicians to take control as policymakers.

Of course, the easiest way to take control of policies would be to assume an administrative position and use your wealth of expertise to promote better policy directions. But this is not the only way you can take charge. There are numerous ways you can advocate by creating favorable policies within your organization and in the community at large. There isn't close to enough space here to list them all, but below I've illustrated two basic and simple ways I hope prove inspirational:

Case 1 - Actions towards changing or making new state-wide or national policies

A Congressman has introduced a bill at the federal level that proposes measures to help women who are socially disadvantaged attend at least 5 prenatal appointments during their pregnancy. You analyze this bill, recognizing its potential impact on the lives of pregnant women and their access to healthcare.

What are some ways you can take charge and make sure the bill sees the light of the day?

There are many ways to express your support of this bill, and ensure it gets discussed seriously.

You can:

- Call this Congressman and express your support, and ask them what ways you can help pass the bill within the confines of professional ethics.
- You can also call your own state representatives and explain why they should support this bill. You can offer evidence-based reasons such as statistics of how many pregnant women do not have access to prenatal care due to being disadvantaged in one way or the other.
- The media is a powerful tool. It can build and it can destroy. Being an expert or authority figure in healthcare, you can write an op-ed on the importance of this bill in your local paper or online.

Case 2 - Actions towards changing or making new organization level policies.

Imagine one of your pregnant female patients does not own a car, and relies on public transportation to find her way to your hospital. She almost never shows up on time for appointments and complains that the

hospital shuttle from the bus stop only comes once an hour.
What are some policy directions you could promote to advocate for your patient?
You can:
- Analyze the shuttle's schedule and set up a meeting with the hospital administrators to discuss the hospital shuttle schedule and how it can be improved.
- If she has consented, you can share her story and advocate for more frequent pick up times during busy clinic hours.
- This could benefit not just this patient but many others, and increase access to healthcare in the local community.

NOTES

CHAPTER 3

PHYSICIANS AS RESEARCHERS

As a physician, you can save one life at a time practicing at your ward, but you can save a million more with just a single research paper.

Research is undeniably the lifeblood of medical advancement. Essentially every drug, therapy, diagnostic tool or form of treatment in modern medicine originated in research. One of the best ways physicians can have a far-reaching impact is by doing research. Despite how far the world has gone in terms of medical advancement, no matter how much we know, there's always more to be discovered in any medical field. The whole point of research is to discover those things that have not yet been discovered, to know things that have not been previously known. The contribution you make by taking part in research can be critical in helping not just the next patient that shows up at your hospital, but people all around the world. Most would agree that the highest potential of clinical research is unlikely to be reached without greater involvement of physicians.

HOW TO DEVELOP INTEREST IN RESEARCH

All scientists are physicians. Our medical curriculum conditions us to think scientifically. A scientist usually formulates a hypothesis, conducts tests on the hypothesis, and thus formulates a plausible conclusion based on accumulated evidence. Similarly, as physicians in daily practice, we sift through and try to make sense of information provided by the patient through interviews, physical examinations, and laboratory tests to identify a problem and devise a treatment plan. Both scientists and physicians share the common task of making sense of otherwise obscure data. This means, as physicians we already possess most of what is needed to be researchers, we just need a little push to get there. During the formative stage of our education, we are introduced to research; but making this a habit and keeping it up during our careers requires both individual, organizational, and political efforts. Individually, there numerous ways physicians can develop interest in research, all beyond the scope of this book. However, we can discuss a few key, constructive ways.

IDENTIFY AN AREA OF INTEREST OR SOMETHING THAT PERSONALLY AFFECTS YOU

Since research is not restricted to any specific medical field, as physicians, we should first endeavor to identify our areas of interest. It's hard enough to join the research-centric community; attempts to foster research interest in an area you consider less interesting is a surefire way to lose motivation. To develop an interest in research, you'll need to first research your area of interest. You might need to identify something that affects you, the health of your patients, or your community, either directly or indirectly. You'll likely foster greater passion for research if the topic has the potential to solve your personal problems, or those of your patients or immediate community. It may all sound a little self-centered, but sometimes, that's just the natural order of things.

For instance, as an oral health professional with a child who has a recurrent oral health problem, your interest in research in the relevant oral health field might certainly be intense and non-relenting. If a solution is achieved through your research, it may save your child, and may perhaps also save millions of other children, too.

IDENTIFY AND JOIN ACTIVE RESEARCH NETWORKS

For most medical fields, there are probably plenty of research groups and individual researchers connected to your topic of interest. There's a huge number of research groups all over the world with dedicated researchers willing to share ideas and experiences. Interacting with people who share their own victories in research can greatly inspire you and significantly heighten your interest towards research in the process. More experienced researchers in your groups or network may be willing to offer valuable advice on your research interest, or point you to good resources. This is an excellent way to keep the fire of your interest burning.

GET A RESEARCH MENTOR

If you have any tiny bit of passion to research, getting a research mentor can help grow that passion. Remember, other people's passion and interest can be contagious. With a mentor who is grounded in, or has great passion for, your area of interest, you'll be able to learn from their expertise. They can share areas within your interest that are unexplored and offer ideas for research directions that would be of value to people in your community, country, or even worldwide.

EXPLORE NEW (AND MORE!) PROBLEMS

No matter how advanced and sophisticated the state-of-the-art has become in any medical field, there's always a problem, and there are always things that could be done to improve them. Even with the breakthrough in malaria treatments, cancer, stem cell, and much more, there are still knowledge gaps that could be plugged, with the potential to save lives. Taking on a research problem with the potential to impact change on a larger scale can be deeply motivating, and a good way to start off developing interest in research. Artificial intelligence and innovation is another raw area waiting to be explored in healthcare.

However, developing interest in research is not just an individual responsibility. Lack of research interest among physicians is usually linked to two important factors: the absence of supportive infrastructures and a lack of facilitating research culture. Organizations and policymakers must change the status quo or influence decisions, policies, and even the physical and social environment to favor research. Research-minded physicians are to a considerable extent a function of their physical, social, and political environment. To encourage physician participation in research, relevant organizational and operational infrastructure needs to be strengthened. Indeed, the entire physician-researcher ecosystem needs to be empowered. This should be done by developing healthy and effective relationships between the encompassing process, structures, and outcomes of research planning and management process. Without doubt, an effective operational and organizational structure is a potent natural catalyst to encourage physician participation in research.

In terms of resources, financial incentives have proven to be an invaluable motivation to encourage research by physicians. Research doesn't come cheap. The instruments, data gathering, travelling - it all weighs heavily on a researcher's pocket. Ethics aside, for some researchers, the motivation to "earn profit" can come into play, primarily to offset the cost of research. But for us as physicians, research could just be a strategic social investment with no idea of immediate reimbursement. Financial incentives must then be weighed by relevant authorities as a potential tool to stimulate interest among prospective physician researchers.

It's true that physicians are trained on research (to some extent) during their education. But such training is almost always not enough. It's necessary for physicians to be further and adequately trained in research methodology and biostatistics to better develop their research skills on core clinical knowledge.

Promotion of research fellowships, mentoring programs, and workshops/seminars designed for physicians can foster better understanding of research, and also provide opportunities to work with research groups and prominent research figures to discuss the practical issues of doing research. Measures should be put in place to introduce research methodology in undergraduate education, postdoctoral training, and even career awards. Health-centric educational institutions need to analyze current practices of research, and reflect upon the possible changes needed to develop a research-focused curriculum.

In the same vein, it's important to rectify the idea that most physicians simply don't want to take part in research: this is not true. Studies have shown that physicians are indeed eager to participate in research, but are obstructed by lack of adequate infrastructures and an inhibiting environment. In order to encourage the participation of more physicians in research, we need to prioritize research and value evidence-based practice. On an organizational level, regular feedback and technical support along with financial compensation are obvious ways to motivate physicians to participate in clinical research.

WHY ALL PHYSICIANS SHOULD BE RESEARCHERS

Medical Research and improved clinical care go hand in hand, and physicians who are at the forefront of research in their respective fields can be confident of providing their patients the best care available.

All physicians are responsible for evaluating their own practice, and there's no better way to do that in a than by using research as a tool. As physicians, we all also need to possess the ability to critically review research done by others. Just as foot soldiers in the frontline are in the best position to understand first-hand the effectiveness of military research on weapons and tactics, so are physicians better positioned to analyze the effectiveness of existing medical care.

Taking part in research enables physicians to evaluate their practice objectively and be directly involved in advancing their discipline. There are many skills to be learnt, potentially making any physician significantly better in their field. Healthcare would definitely benefit from a research-engaged physician workforce. Research projects would focus more closely on patient priorities, meaning the available and often limited research resources would be channeled to the right areas.

As long as physicians remain at the forefront of medical innovations by participating in research, their patients would also be able to gain access to cutting-edge medicine. Physicians would become better versed in the relevant literature of their field, and develop transferable skills and enquiring minds. From involvement in medical advancement to participation in quality improvement, research introduces a richness and dynamism to any physician's medical career.

Physicians' participation in research is essential in ensuring that the knowledge of the causes and treatments of disease are up to date. It's essential in designing new treatments and ways of working with the aim of improving the health and quality of life of patients.

Clinical experiences and interacting directly with patients can give physicians a unique and alternative perspective on the direction that research efforts should be focused, in order to benefit patients the most. Physicians' participation in research can give them great insight into how new breakthroughs can be best translated to be of practical benefit to patients. Being researchers offers physicians a unique opportunity to ask immediately pertinent questions that are the most relevant for the direct improvement of patient care. Since they work face to face with patients, they encounter more relevant factors, including the tiniest of details that could be critical to a patient's survival but would be otherwise obscured or not considered by normal researchers.

Going back to our military analogy: foot soldiers using a new bulletproof vest developed as a result of research may notice that while the new vest offers better protection, it's a bit heavier and reduces a soldier's maneuverability. In this case, this could be a mission critical, lifesaving detail, otherwise obscured during the research and development phase. Similarly, in medical research, there are some lifesaving, treatment-critical details which are only revealed through practical experience. It's critically important that physicians play a role in the medical research processes, and that research is not considered solely the responsibility of academic scientists.

Different studies have provided evidence that patients who receive medical care in research-active institutions have better outcomes than those in less research-centric institutions. These patients are more likely to benefit from earlier access to new treatments, latest technologies, and improved approaches to medical care.

As physicians venturing into the research domain; whether you're contributing to large collaborative projects, recruiting patients into other researchers' trials, or contributing to quality improvement or any form of research in anyway - your seemingly trivial actions hold the potential to effect enormous positive changes.

An important sub-domain in biomedical research is clinical and translational research, which establishes the effectiveness of drugs or treatment techniques on patients. This is usually carried out in the form of clinical trials. Physicians are an invaluable asset in clinical trials. Since they're viewed as lifesavers, they receive lots of love and respect in their communities, especially from individuals they've provided health care to. Over time, they build strong bonds with individuals in the community as they help to deliver babies and treat sick loved ones. Physicians are thus admired and trusted within a population. It then becomes easier for them (compared to full time medical researchers) to recruit patients who meet certain criteria for clinical trials.

It's important to emphasize the two most important things that make physicians uniquely well-positioned to contribute to research and ensure that medical advances are patient-centric. First, we maintain regular clinical contact with patients which makes us better able to observe patterns and identify the research needs that make the most difference to patients. Secondly, our understanding of what is realistically translatable into everyday practice enables research findings to be realized and implemented in a way that will be most effective for people. It's clear that physicians need to remain actively involved in research at all levels.

THE IMPACT OF RESEARCH ON PHYSICIANS

There's a substantial amount of evidence that points to the impact of research on physicians. Firstly, research has immensely equipped physicians with vital and current information about disease trends and risk factors, possible outcomes of treatment, and best patterns of medical care. As physicians, research is necessary for us to continuously question our clinical practice and reduce complacency. It helps us to deploy better ways of doing things. Without scientific investigations in research, advancement in medical practice would stagnate.

While it may be impossible to really quantify the impact of research on physicians, it's important to nonetheless analyze the impact of physicians' participation in research. Many great intellectuals have argued that research and medical practice should not and cannot be mixed productively. Paul De Kruif devotes entire chapters in his book "*Our Medicine Men Trying*" to explain that research and medical practice shouldn't be attempted simultaneously by a physician. He claims, "It is certain that this pretense of physicians threatens to turn medicine from its primordial and proper function of healing and soothing our ills, toward a quackish assumption of the dignity of science. It is possible to study disease scientifically, but it is absurd to presume that this can be done by the rank and file of doctors." Paul De Kruif was not alone in his assertions; other intellectuals have made similar assertions. Though a great number of physicians and scientists, including myself, would easily dismiss such assertions today, their views still pose a pertinent and important question that discourages the involvement of some doctors in actively pursuing a research role.

Despite Paul De Kruif's views, can the roles of scientist and physician be efficiently balanced? Does the result of their involvement in science have significant impact on a physician's medical practice? As we will soon see, medical practice and scientific research can indeed coexist. The shared characteristics of both a scientist and a physician can certainly be utilized in scientific investigations in ways that can significantly improve medical care. It's important to consider the impact of physicians' participation in research if we are to encourage more physician involvement.

Theobald Smith is an example of a physician that exemplifies the impact of research on physicians and clinical practice as a whole. After graduating from Albany Medical College in 1884, his clinical experience proved to be quite useful in his research into the "Texas Fever" that devastated livestock across the country. Texas fever was very problematic and presented a rather puzzling challenge to livestock farmers of the time. He noticed that southern cows which were brought into contact with northern cows died mysteriously. The southern cows would fall extremely sick just a short while after establishing contact with northern cows, and no medication available at the time could help the cows once they fell sick. This problem occurred irrespective of whether the southern cows were brought to the northern environment or the northern cows were brought to the southern environment. The southern cows just didn't stand any survival chance, as long as they were brought in close proximity to the northern cows.

Dr. Smith took on the task of researching the puzzling problem, an idea that was generally scoffed at during the time. The cattlemen suggested that ticks could be the cause of the problem, but the idea that insects could transmit or cause disease was an absurdity at the time. Nobody was really convinced that ticks could be responsible for the mysterious phenomenon. But Smith believed otherwise. In what was probably the first in a series of studies to prove that insects could indeed cause diseases, Dr. Smith set out to test his hypothesis.

Using an effective experimental technique, Smith created different experimental groups by putting different cows in separate fields. He introduced the ticks from the southern cows to the northern cows and observed tick dispersion, and repeated the same for the southern cows. As a by-product of the research, his experiments brought much insight into how ticks live and thrive off their host, something that was generally unknown at the time. It also produced insights into another less understood medical concept at that time:

immunity. His research was able to unravel more mysteries about immunity, giving it a medical explanation rather than the common superstitions of the time. However, perhaps most importantly, his conclusions after his experiments was that insects could indeedcause or transmit diseases, and ticks were causing the cows' illness in this case.

His research helped to establish the link between parasitic insects and disease. Subsequently, the full impact of his research could then be evidenced in establishing the causes of diseases such as malaria, yellow fever, and Lyme disease. It was then relatively easy to decipher the causes of diseases whenever parasitic insects were involved. The result of his research has since spread across different frontiers in medicine and hugely impacted clinical practice and multiple medical sciences. Dr. Smith's sound research has greatly benefitted the medical profession, cementing the importance and value of physicians' participation in research.

Another noteworthy physician in this respect is Dr. Judah Folkman. An excellent surgeon by the standards of his time, he was chief of surgery of Children's Hospital Boston for fourteen years. Throughout his service at the hospital, he was immersed in the theory of tumor angiogenesis, a radically new idea for the time. He was very confident he could use this theory against cancer. Many doubted and questioned his devotion to his patients in need of surgery since he spent a great deal of time on research. But according to his biography authored by Robert Cooke, Dr. Folkman was actually able to serve his patients more effectively as a result of continued research in this domain. His successes in angiogenesis greatly impacted his medical practice. His ability to constantly pose serious questions and solve persistent problems in medical practice made him an excellent physician by all accounts, even by today's standard. Although his dedication to research far exceeds that of today's average physician researchers, he shows us that physician participation in research could positively impact both medical practice and scientific knowledge.

Another notable illustration is that made by the physician David Weatherall. In his book on the role of medical research in healthcare, *Science and the Quiet Art: The Role of Medical Research in Health Care*, Weatherall makes an important illustration using appendicitis. Since there is still no standardized or definitive diagnostic test for appendicitis, there's great reliance on a physician's diagnostic skill, observations, and previous insights garnered from practical experience. The participation of experienced physicians on identifying appendicitis is extremely valuable.

Medicine has always been an "art," but with increased participation in medical research, we can come even closer to steering medical practice away from mere empiricism to a true scientific discipline. Exemplary physician researchers like Dr. Smith and Dr. Folkman have proven that research and medical practice can indeed coexist to fight disease and improve healthcare systems. Medical research has had enormous impact on medical practice and its role can be best described as multifaceted, since it not only improves and facilitate medical practice for physicians, but educates them as well. Research has helped physicians understand the true complexities of the diseases they face in practice. Greater knowledge on diseases has helped physicians better target disease, reducing premature death and improving general quality of life. As the reputable Lewis Thomas put it succinctly in the final pages of his book, *The Medusa and the Snail*: "We need to know more ... We have discovered how to ask important questions, and now we really do need, as an urgent matter, for the sake of our civilization, to obtain some answers. We now know that we cannot do this any longer by searching our minds, for there is not enough there to search, nor can we find the truth by guessing at it or by making up stories for ourselves. We cannot stop where we are, stuck with today's level of understanding, nor can we go back ... We need science, more and better science, not for its technology, not for leisure, not even for health or longevity, but for the hope of wisdom which our kind of culture must acquire for its survival."

BENEFITS AND DOWNSIDES OF DOING RESEARCH – PERSONAL AND PROFESSIONAL LEVEL

Research greatly benefits any participating physician, but it also has its burdens. Just like every other thing in life, research has its pros and cons. For the purpose of this book, we'll consider its benefits and downsides both on the professional and the personal level.

THE BENEFITS

On a personal level, one of the greatest benefits of research to a physician is personal satisfaction. The joy that comes from knowing you're at the forefront of medical advancement and that you're contributing your part to the science of medicine as well as the art. There's a satisfaction in knowing you've been able to objectively question, evaluate, and test different approaches in medical research and practice in ways that could potentially benefit humankind. Pause for a while and think of the feeling of achievement, joy, and pride in service to humankind gained by those researchers who developed polio vaccines, chemotherapy for cancer, or drugs for managing HIV/AIDS. As a physician, the joy of saving a life in your ward is immense, but the immense joy of saving potentially thousands cannot be overstated.

On the professional side, as a physician-researcher, you're considered an important figure in health research and indeed healthcare in general. You become invaluable in patient-oriented research. Your small contribution helps in expanding the knowledge base of medicine and affords you the opportunity to offer patients the best in cutting-edge medical care. Your participation in research also opens your eyes to a broad range of medical innovation, satisfies your intellectual curiosity, and perhaps very importantly assists in career advancement. Your participation in research may add prestige to your practice or institution. It's often understood that the field of medical research would stagnate without the participation of researchers with clinical experience with the health conditions and service systems being researched.

THE DOWNSIDES

As physicians participating in research, there's bound to be some form of "role confusion," both external and internal. External role confusion comes from not being able to clearly explain to others what you really do. Internal role confusion on the other hand comes primarily from the fact that research and actual day-to-day medical practice consist of fundamentally different tasks in the work environment, including things like work location, schedule, and perhaps even professional attire. While research is typically less rigid in this regard, clinical practice could be much stricter. A physician-researcher who alternates between these two professional identities may experience challenges adjusting. Although some physicians may find switching roles fun and exciting, a lot more will find themselves conflicted about their professional identity. This identity confusion may cause a physician-researcher to gravitate toward the work role that they're most comfortable with, and may be tempted to withdraw from either commitment.

Furthermore, different discussions on research ethics highlight a potential conflict of interest between participants and the scientific aims of the study. Since clinical research and trials would normally involve human subjects, it may be inevitable for a physician-researcher to experience an internal clash between the need to act in the patient's best interest and the scientific mandate to pursue truth with appropriate rigor. This usually results in a situation where participants in clinical research wrongly assume that the goal of clinical research is therapeutic or remedial. This means that participants don't understand, for example, that the "clinical activity" they're taking part in may not necessarily treat or heal them of any ailment, and that they're randomly assigned to a study condition that may not be in their best personal interest. As we discussed earlier, physicians form a strong bound with individuals and families, so this misconception is even more likely to occur if the study investigator is a physician that participants know, respect, and trust as a treatment provider.

HOW TO JUGGLE THE RESEARCH AND CLINICAL ASPECTS OF A PHYSICIAN'S WORKING LIFE

Establishing a balance between everyday clinical practice and research work is a challenging task. These challenges often vary depending on the demands of both your clinical and research roles and how interrelated these roles may be. Considering this, it's safe to say that it's probably easier to juggle clinical work and research work if your research is more "clinical" than lab-based. But biomedical research can be diverse and this may not always be the case. Physician-researchers can take part in either Basic research, Medical education research, Health service improvement research, Translational research, Epidemiological research or clinical research.

The challenges can also lie in figuring out how to deal with the urgency of immediate patient-related work versus trying to meet deadlines for grant applications, or trying to write research papers when also doing day-to-day clinical work with difficult shift schedules. Nonetheless, many physicians have successfully been able to juggle the two roles. Let's consider some important factors that might contribute to this success.

EFFECTIVE TIME MANAGEMENT AND ORGANIZATIONAL SKILLS

One of the most important ingredients for successfully juggling the two roles is excellent time management and organization. This is necessary to efficiently use the available time and effort. As a physician, you're probably already running a tight schedule, so introducing a research role into the mix can be a recipe for disaster if not properly managed. It's essential to be clear about the time available to fulfill the demands placed on us from both roles. As physician-researchers, we need to set clear, specific, and feasible objectives. The key is designing an efficient schedule that accommodates both roles according to their perceived time requirements. Adjust this time schedule gradually as you adapt to both roles to reflect a plausible time frame to get work done. Also, when presented with any opportunity in either role, always try to evaluate its potential impact on the time left for the other role.

EFFECTIVE PROFESSIONAL COMMUNICATION

It's quite important as physician-researchers to communicate appropriately with others about the two worlds we find ourselves. Depending on your research role, many of your work colleagues may not understand what you do on a day-to-day basis, or what should be expected of you. It's quite useful to talk about both sides of the job, to take away some of the mystery surrounding what we do. This helps work colleagues understand the pressures we face, and eases external pressure, respecting both sides of your work as well as making it clear to everyone exactly what you're up to.

MENTORSHIP

Mentorship from established physician-researchers is quite useful in striking a balance between the world of clinical work and research. Find a mentor who appreciates both your roles and who has successfully juggled them themselves. This means they can provide you with useful advice on how they deal with both clinical work and research demands. Mentors are in a good position to help ensure that your objectives are appropriate, and they may even help you explain what you need to prioritize to get the best out of both worlds.

AVOIDING FEELINGS OF INFERIORITY IN EITHER ROLE

In the beginning, there's bound to be a feeling of slight inferiority in either role. Physician-researchers are likely to feel like less of an expert in one or the other arena, than those who focus all their time on just one. Part of this usually comes from the fact that it's challenging to keep up with the latest developments and literatures from both sides. It's reasonable to accept the possibility of being less than perfect in either role, but feelings of inferiority should not be seriously entertained.

It might seem daunting at first, but even with a seemingly impossible schedule, physicians can develop creative ways to manage their participation in medical practice and scientific investigations. It's more than possible for physicians to juggle their dedication to individual patients with a dedication to research aimed at improving the health of entire populations.

Chapter 4

PHYSICIANS AS ADMINISTRATORS

Healthcare is a complex machine. It gets even more complex with each passing day. There's an ever-increasing need to find a balance between quality and cost, as well as between technology and humanity. There are always competing needs, both of which are usually critical to healthcare delivery. There are always challenges in prioritizing one need at the expense of the other. Tackling these challenges requires extraordinary leaders, i.e those who know just enough of what should be sacrificed of one to support the other. It requires leaders who can strike a plausible balance between two often competing needs.

As physicians, we were introduced to the language of medicine both in its crude and modern form. We spent our formative days getting used to its Latin and Greek roots, its abbreviations and its acronyms, and today we communicate effectively with other physicians because of it. But during this time, we failed to learn the language used in the "business of healthcare." For most of us, this was never a problem, since the "system" didn't need it, our curriculum didn't include it, and we didn't personally notice its absence.

Unfortunately, the healthcare landscape has since rapidly evolved, and more than ever physicians need to be grounded in the "business of healthcare" and its language. Before things started evolving at such a rapid pace, healthcare was different. Physicians primarily provided medical care to patients, business managers then managed the physicians, and business executives and administrators then ran the entire hospital. This separation of responsibilities initially made sense. Physicians - dentists, pediatricians, optometrists, surgeons, and all medical care givers - needed to stick strictly to what they did best: offering medical care. The managers and the powers that be ran the hospitals and had fancy degrees in business economics and needed to be in charge of everything else. However, this delineation resulted in the creation of a silo effect in health care, with each party focusing solely on its own division and responsibilities within the system, often at the expense of efficiencies in other divisions. This usually led to several conflicts of interest and a great deal of mistrust in the system.

The system has evolved, and the language used in the business of healthcare has also evolved to now include administrative and managerial lexicons. The trends have changed, and it's no safe for a dichotomy to exist in the healthcare system. There's an even greater need for reconciliation between the role of care giving and administration. There needs to be some form of convergence of these roles. Unfortunately, just as most hospital administrators lack valuable insight on practical care giving, most physicians are depressively deficient in the administrative skills needed to provide leadership in the business of healthcare.

Physicians generally possess the skills for clinical care, and managers only the skills for administering the business of health care. Physicians who can affect a convergence — through natural talent or additional leadership training — are better positioned to lead health care organizations as physician-executives. Physicians occupying managerial, administrative or executive positions offer enormous rewards both in personal professional satisfaction and in organizational success.

CLINICAL AND ADMINISTRATIVE ROLES

In an organizational setting, clinical and administrative roles are differently and uniquely structured but nonetheless equally important. Clinical roles encompass all the day-to-day medical and care giving practice of physicians. It includes everything from interviewing patients and diagnosis to surgery and therapy, plus a wide range of therapeutic responsibilities. An administrative role in the other hand encompasses responsibilities ranging from formulation of organization-level policies to overall financial and personnel management of a medical establishment. In most medical organizations, these responsibilities are limited to purely administrative activities, with occupiers of administrative positions having little to no contact with actual patients. The main aim of this role is to centrally coordinate all facets of healthcare delivery. Clinicians and hospital admins have traditionally been at loggerheads, due these conflicting interests.

In today's world, there's a greater need for synergy between the two roles. Physicians were once assumed to be ill-prepared for administrative roles. Their training molded them to become patient-centered cogs in the healthcare machine, with little to no understanding of the bigger picture. However, things are changing. The need for improvement in healthcare delivery now requires patient-centered leadership. Physicians participating in both clinical and administrative roles are uniquely positioned to identify both business and clinical needs of organizations.

THE RISE OF THE HOSPITAL ADMINISTRATOR

Recently, hospital administrators have dominated healthcare, and this has had an enormous effect on medical practice, further complicating the entire healthcare landscape. Today's medicine has certainly skewed more towards business, and physicians that are grounded in business as physician-administrators are much more successful. There is undoubtedly a role for administrators in the system, since they're still necessary for coordination and offering support to the clinical work of physicians. Complexities related to human resources, staffing, regulations, compliance, and other activities calls for administrators. However, their role in efficient healthcare delivery has quickly become a problem.

Administrators who mostly have zero relevant clinical knowledge or experience have evolved into overlords of medical practice. Even with such a deficiency, they're thrust into positions where they dictate how physicians should work, when to work, and where to work. Creativity, which is an important feature of medical practice, has become greatly suppressed and frowned upon by administrators. There's now a primarily protocol-based system, where physicians have to almost always strictly follow "protocols and algorithms." Physicians are fast becoming worker bees in the vast factory of the administrators. The evolution of healthcare towards an administrator-driven practice has pushed medicine even further away from patient-centered leadership. Money and cost-cutting is the major driver. Physicians are no more valued in the system because they have different opinions honed from practical experience, which administrators consider financially unviable.

Administrators just want to run a business; they want to meet targets, the want to reel it in big time. This is usually at the expense of efficiency and generally improved healthcare. Administrative cost more than anything else is now sky high, and it seems the "talkers" are gradually not just dictating but also earning more than the "doers." Further compounding the complexity of the administrator-physician debacle is that physicians develop intense scientific discipline as part of their training. This usually inculcates in them the value of autonomous decision-making, personal achievement, and improvement as against that of any institution. Healthcare organizations have generally fallen behind and are just recently becoming aware of the importance of developing leaders with a practical clinical experience – or, put simply, physician leaders.

A CALL TO ACTION - WHAT PHYSICIANS MUST DO

As physicians we must take a stand. The status quo has not just become unfavorable to us as physicians, but has badly affected the core product of healthcare, i.e. the patient-physician relationship. We must passionately advocate for our patients and for our profession. Medicine is bound to stagnate, and become devoid of innovation in clinical practice without committed, caring, and compassionate physicians being allowed to practice medicine and assume leadership roles. Physicians must wrestle back control of healthcare and limit the power of hospital administrators. The many challenges facing healthcare today call for strong, authentic leadership - and physicians are uniquely positioned to assume such leadership.

As healthcare professionals, we're in the middle of one of the most dynamic periods in healthcare history. The healthcare industry is moving at a pace few are able to keep up with. Unfortunately, the relationship between those who actually deliver medical care and those who are responsible for the administration of the entire healthcare machine has never been more fractured, tense, or challenged. It has never been more complicated because at the basic level, physicians and administrators have traditionally not trusted each other.

If physicians must fix the problems, they must urgently learn the modern business of healthcare. A great number of physicians complete their training with little or no understanding of administration, financing or organization of healthcare. This is unfortunately a huge limitation, it's no wonder there is sometimes deep suspicion between those administering healthcare and physicians. However, this doesn't necessarily mean that administrators are always on the right side but merely misunderstood. Administrators are a substantial part of the problem in the system, but as physicians who clamor for better healthcare, we must educate ourselves about the administration and financing of healthcare. Unfortunately, as noted earlier, physicians do not get comprehensive education on healthcare policies, administration, finance or organization during their entire premedical education, medical school, residency or fellowship.

Physicians must educate themselves on these pertinent issues. Education opportunities abound for physicians who want to make a shift towards administration. There are also different opportunities for physicians to enter the administrative realm of healthcare. Consider for example the number of adverts for physician-executive positions in professional journals, and of course the rapid increase in seminars/workshops specifically designed to train physician leaders.

As a matter of fact, studies have shown that physician-run hospitals are more likely to score higher in general quality of care and patient-oriented health service delivery than manager-run hospitals. Of course, the results of these studies don't necessarily prove that doctors make better leaders, but they're certainly consistent with that claim. Support for the value of medically experienced administrators in healthcare can also be observed in other sectors. For instance, scholar-administrators have helped to better enhance research outputs in educational institutions. In sports, basketball teams with coaches who were former players themselves have been linked to improved chances of success. Similarly, in Formula One Racing, former drivers have particularly excelled as team leaders. In general, industry or domain experts have always been linked with better organizational performance.

It can be argued that, when physicians are leaders in health care, they're armed with credible insights as to the requirements of their "fellow physicians" for better healthcare service delivery. They're better informed through a shared understanding about the motivations of healthcare providers. Since most physicians spend their careers looking at things with a patient-focused perspective, physicians moving into executive positions are better suited to striking a balance between organization-focused and patient-focused strategy and policies.

Thanks to their wealth of practical experience, physicians usually know what's required to complete a job to the highest standard. They're therefore more likely to "go beyond" to create the right working environment to achieve those required standards. They're better suited to set appropriate and feasible goals, as well as accurately evaluate everyone's contributions. Fortunately, some healthcare and medical institutions are fast realizing that the mix of knowledge and skills that physicians introduce to administration can spur enormous improvement and great organizational change.

Physician-administrators appear to be the quite effective leaders precisely because they are physicians. Yet, leadership in healthcare requires much more than just being physicians; it requires great leadership and social skills. All in all, physicians must get themselves accustomed to the fundamental principles of business, at least within the realms of healthcare delivery. They must strive for personal leadership development to be even better positioned for administration. They must clamor in the interest of future physicians, and for the integration of administrative skills training into formal medical curricula.

NOTES

Chapter 5

PHYSICIANS AS ENTREPRENEURS

According to conventional wisdom, doctors are lousy entrepreneurs and no better as businesspeople. This line of reasoning holds that they should just stick to caring for patients and leave the entrepreneurial and business part to others. Considering that a physician's training does not encourage entrepreneurial skills, this line of thinking is plausible to some extent, but not necessarily true. Most importantly, in today's healthcare landscape and economy in general, these beliefs, no matter how justified, are no longer sustainable if physicians are to thrive. Rather, it's important to focus on the fact that physicians do have the potential to make great entrepreneurs. Admittedly, only a small percentage of practicing physicians have entrepreneurial and innovation mindsets, but just a few would be enough to disrupt the system and add substantial value. However, as physicians, we were never trained in anything other than being good physicians. The reality is that, to a great extent, we're still stuck in the webs of the old system.

In the old system, physicians were taught to muscle it through medical school, push pass residency, get a "good job" and prudently work our way to retirement. Then we would gratefully take the pensions and like a fairy tale, we would "live happily ever after." Or better still, we could work till we drop, while still priding ourselves on being "good physicians." Today, however, things have changed drastically. It's no longer good enough to just be "a good physician" as our sole professional identify. However, because we are still partly stuck in webs of the past, being a physician *and* an entrepreneur is foreign to most of us. Nonetheless, with the proper mindset, vision, and skills, we can break the chains that the current medical system has shackled us with, and establish ourselves as competent physicians-entrepreneurs.

In this chapter, we'll present valuable insights about the need for entrepreneurship, what it entails, and myths and tips for physician-entrepreneurs.

WHAT IS A PHYSICIAN ENTREPRENEUR?

The definition of a physician-entrepreneur is broad and often results in misconceptions and myths. There is some sort of mysterious cloud of confusion surrounding what a physician entrepreneur is, and what it entails. We'll walk through the whole idea while dissecting its subcomponents.

Briefly, we can define entrepreneurship as the pursuit of opportunity with scarce, uncontrolled resources. It's widely defined as the entire process between designing, launching, and running a business while taking on a greater than normal financial risk. In the context of healthcare, entrepreneurship is not much different. The ultimate goal of all entrepreneurs, including physician entrepreneurs, is to create value by solving a problem through the deployment of innovation. Both physicians and entrepreneurs are inherently problem solvers: it's definitely not a secret that there are enormous problems to solve in health care. With this definition, physician-entrepreneurs are health professionals who make conscious efforts to solve a problem in healthcare, while often taking on financial risk with possible options for reimbursement.

In the US, healthcare amounts to about 18% of the GDP and is rising with no signs of stopping. Everyone who cares wants to cut down on healthcare spending - business owners, politicians, private individuals, everyone. We all want the best in health care, but nobody is willing to go bankrupt to get it. Unlike the trend in other science and technology industry, rather than decreasing, the cost of drug is rapidly increasing with time. I remember one of my last patients in clinic one day was a charming 82-year old gentleman who'd had a stroke a year earlier due to atrial fibrillation (an irregular heart rhythm). He was recovering. At one point during our conversation he said something that has stuck with me ever since. He told me that he only had $25 in his wallet and, rather than spend it on the medication he needed (apixaban) he decided he'd use it to buy coffee at Starbucks for his wife when he went to meet her later that day at her nursing home, where she was recovering from a hip fracture. This was a man who knew full well the consequences of not taking his medication. Whenever I hear people talk about curbing healthcare spending, I think of this elderly man and his wife.

The problems in our present healthcare reality are enormous and to some extent, we can say physician-entrepreneurs are those health professionals that take a step out of the system in other to solve these problems. Don't misunderstand me; "stepping out of the system" doesn't necessarily mean the same thing as private practice, nor is it fundamentally about practice management. There are surely different roles for physician-entrepreneurs to fill, including those of small to medium sized business owners, technopreneurs, and social entrepreneurs. But employed physicians can still be physician-entrepreneurs.

In this capacity they're better referred to as *intrapreneurs*, which entails an employed physician acting in an entrepreneurial role as freelancers, consultants or physician investors. Just like their colleagues in independent practice, intrapreneurs have as much potential to be entrepreneurial. Learning programming, coding, and enlightening ourselves on artificial intelligence (AI) to integrate technology into medical practice is an attractive arena that has certainly kept me interested. In most people's opinion, this is the next big thing waiting to happen in healthcare. Amazon and other tech giants are currently in the brainstorming phase, but inevitably, this miracle in waiting is just a matter of time.

I heard the CEO of Google/Alphabet, Mr. Sunder Pichai, explaining some of the fascinating initiatives by these IT companies in the healthcare arena. One example is the fact that Google analyzes big data with a predictive model for readmission (admittedly, it's funny to hear about de-identification and data privacy from companies like these, but nevertheless). Similarly, the diabetic retinopathy screening data of millions of patients were being looked into to identify high risk of heart attack and stroke in patients. With these issues, timely intervention could spare patients serious disability. Admittedly this is a field in its infancy, but I believe the penetration of IT companies into healthcare is inevitable. Physicians need to familiarize themselves with coding, big data mining and artificial intelligence *now*, to ensure they're poised to respond to these advancements as they happen.

Physician-entrepreneurs have a good knowledge of the problems of the system, and can leverage this knowledge to create value for people in ways other than giving direct medical care. Every existing threat to medical practice represents an important opportunity for physician-entrepreneurs to create value by solving a problem. Every industrialized nation is continuously faced with the challenge of providing their population with adequate health services using often scarce resources. Innovation and physician entrepreneurship is the bridge that is gradually ameliorating this enormous problem.

PHYSICIAN-ENTREPRENEURS AS ENTREPRENEURS

In this context, "physician entrepreneurs as entrepreneurs" refers to physician entrepreneurs who are self-employed or under independent practice.

Physician entrepreneurship opens up self-employment opportunities for physicians, enabling them to use innovative approaches to pursue their personal dreams while improving health outcomes. Like other entrepreneurs, a physician-entrepreneur is generally considered to be a proprietor of a business which offers services related to healthcare, being it direct care, research, administrative, educational, or consultative in nature. This means the physician is self-employed and is directly accountable to the client for whom they provide those services. These physicians may conduct private clinical practice, own a business or run an education or research consultancy. Thus, physician-entrepreneurs as entrepreneurs are unique innovators who make initiatives that lead to change or improvement of health systems. They independently participate in innovations in healthcare, which directly improve health outcomes, lead to better diagnosis and treatment options, as well as improve general efficiency and cost effectiveness within the healthcare system.

The fundamental characteristics of entrepreneurship include using individual creativity to develop new ideas, as well as the improvement of services and their delivery. It also includes creative design of new products or ways to use existing products. Physician-entrepreneurs as entrepreneurs combine this entrepreneurial characteristic with specialist skills and knowledge in healthcare to develop products and services which they market to external sources.

PHYSICIAN ENTREPRENEURS AS INTRAPRENEURS

Unlike the independent entrepreneur we discussed earlier, a physician intrapreneur is usually a salaried employee, currently working under a healthcare institution like a government run hospital. They design, promote, and deliver innovative health products or services within their employers' institution, and within that organizational framework. The physician and the employer jointly bear the risks and share the benefits. The type of innovations designed by intrapreneurs are usually guided by the need to improve processes or develop valuable new products or services that are within the organizational bounds.

Globally, there's increasing pressure on healthcare systems as nations strive to meet the healthcare needs of their citizens efficiently and economically. We define both physician-entrepreneurs and intrapreneurs as effective tools within the system for bridging innovation gaps in healthcare.

TIPS FOR THE PHYSICIAN ENTREPRENEUR

Like any other social entrepreneur, success doesn't come cheap for a physician-entrepreneur, but the following tips may certainly help.

YOU NEED TO HAVE A CAUSE AND A CLEAR VISION

It's one thing to *start* being a physician entrepreneur but it's another thing to *keep* being one. The consistency and determination needed for success comes from a clear vision. Lots of temptations may come along the way. You may have a conflict of interest with your employer or a big company might offer some huge chunk of money to buy you out. While this may be tempting, your whole vision as a physician-entrepreneur, the problems you set out to solve, and the values you wanted to create may all go down the drain if you fail to maintain you will, determination and a crystal clear vision.

YOU MUST BE WILLING TO TAKE RISKS AS A PHYSICIAN-ENTREPRENEUR

As physicians, we face different kinds of risks as part of our day-to-day medical practice. The ability to understand and efficiently manage risk is critical for success. Any physician-entrepreneur should learn to embrace risks as challenges, and devise creative ways to face them. The whole concept of entrepreneurship rests strongly on the willingness to take calculated risks. The question of whether the risk is worth taking or not is something you need to decide based on your comprehension of the situation.

ALWAYS LISTEN TO YOURSELF

While it's important to take advice from others who have succeeded in similar endeavors, don't be afraid of following your instincts. Don't worry about making a decision even if it's not the most popular choice. As the saying goes, "go with your gut."

BEING A PHYSICIAN-ENTREPRENEUR NEEDS TIME AND METICULOUS PLANNING

If you've spent a chunk of your carrier just being a "physician," making the switch might be a little daunting. You surely shouldn't expect to just set up and get going. Establishing yourself as a physician entrepreneur will take careful planning and years of hard work. In terms of planning, you need to figure out the best time to start up, infrastructural requirements, your source of funds, what to call success, and how you'll deal with the inevitable challenges. Meticulous planning and asking the right questions are important cornerstones to becoming a successful entrepreneur in any field, and it's no different in healthcare.

FINANCIAL EDUCATION IS IMPORTANT

If you want to go far as an entrepreneur, financial expertise is indispensable. Depending on the structure and size of your "innovation," having good knowledge of financing could be critical to your success. You should be willing to open yourself up to the world of financing, even though it's completely different from your everyday medical practice.

FAILURE IS NOT THE END; IT'S THE BEST TEACHER

As you push to reach your entrepreneurial goals, you'll almost certainly fail, many more times than you'd like! But this is quite normal. It happens everywhere: in sports, in arts, or in other scientific fields. This means you shouldn't be afraid of failure. Be prepared for it. When it eventually comes, if you're prepared, you'll overcome it. If you were a little sloppy, then you should admit it and learn for next time. For what it's worth, it helps to see failure as a lesson rather than "failure." Insecurities like fear of failure can kill the entrepreneurial spirit.

EXPOSE YOURSELF TO PHYSICIAN AND NON-PHYSICIAN ENTREPRENEURS

The positive influence you get by surrounding yourself with successful physician-entrepreneurs is contagious. Apart from the doses of motivation and encouragement you get, they may be skilled in areas that you may not be, and can offer valuable advice for your success. Surrounding yourself with successful peers challenges you to succeed. As a matter of fact, networking and connecting with other entrepreneurs is an excellent way to nurture your entrepreneurial skills.

YOU DON'T NEED TO BE A BUSINESS EXPERT OR HAVE AN MBA TO BECOME A PHYSICIAN-ENTREPRENEUR

This is definitely not true. Sure, an MBA and expertise in business is an added advantage, but it's not "can't-do-without" kind of advantage. Since you need some sort of business understanding before stepping into the world of entrepreneurship, you can sign up for a business coaching program or training courses. This is usually enough to give you a good foundation before stepping into the world of entrepreneurship. Besides learning what you'll need to navigate the sometimes complex world of business and entrepreneurship, you already have all you need as a physician.

YOU DON'T NEED A LOT OF DISPOSABLE INCOME TO KICKSTART YOUR ENTREPRENEURIAL PLANS

Another widely believed myth. A lot of physician-entrepreneurs start their businesses with very little capital. Though more money is probably better, how much capital you need depends on what you're trying to do. Nonetheless, if you are new to the whole idea of physician entrepreneurship, try to start small. It might not be the next big thing in medical practice, but it might help save a life next door.

YOU DON'T HAVE TO QUIT YOUR EVERYDAY MEDICAL PRACTICE TO BE A SUCCESSFUL PHYSICIAN-ENTREPRENEUR

You don't have to quit your salaried day job to become a full time physician-entrepreneur in order to succeed. This is the whole origin of the term "intrapreneur." Most physician-entrepreneurs start their ventures while practicing clinical medicine - it's possibly even safer that way. These physician-entrepreneurs continue their everyday medical practice, and consider their entrepreneurial endeavors their "side gig." They sometimes even still continue, when their so-called "side-gig" becomes big enough to be the "main gig." You can absolutely keep wearing your clinical practice hat while growing and promoting your entrepreneurial endeavors.

WHY THE RISING NEED FOR PHYSICIAN-ENTREPRENEURS?

A disruption in health care is inevitable at this point. Better technology and the need for more efficient healthcare will be the major drivers, and entrepreneurship offers physicians a safety net while giving patients improved healthcare options for when this happens.

The threads of healthcare, technology, and business are becoming increasingly interwoven. In today's world, the power of technological innovation in healthcare is greater than ever. Technology has enormously impacted the ways physicians diagnose and administer medical care, and the way they communicate with patients and each other. The rapid infiltration of technology into healthcare has created more opportunities for physicians to pursue career or professional interests outside the bounds of the traditional healthcare institution. Technological changes together with a wide range of challenges creates a rising demand for physician-entrepreneurs. The whole idea of physicians becoming entrepreneurs in healthcare is not entirely new, but it has gradually evolved over time. Modern physician-entrepreneurs have redefined what it means to be a physician, moving past entrepreneurship as just about private practice and more about entrepreneurial ventures way beyond the scope of normal clinical duties.

Recently, physician-entrepreneurs have immersed themselves in medical innovation, positively changing how care is delivered to patients. Their participation is highly sought after in healthcare to help reshape the traditional business model. Physician-entrepreneurs are also increasingly participating in the development of new software and tech devices aimed at improving clinical outcomes for patients. They're energetically and passionately involved in creating solutions due to their frustrations with current healthcare inefficiencies. Some are getting involved because entrepreneurship offers them an opportunity to make a greater impact on patients than would be possible in a normal clinical setting. A considerable number even get involved because of the intellectual stimulation that comes from innovation, while still others are motivated purely by possible financial gain.

Regardless of the motivations behind their involvement in entrepreneurship, a physician's valuable insight into healthcare makes them more than suited for a wide range of important innovations in healthcare. The legacies of early physician-entrepreneurs are still with us today. One notable example is cardiac surgeon Albert Starr. Dr. Starr was affected by rheumatic fever, an ailment that causes the narrowing of the heart valves with a marked predominance for mitral valve involvement The absence of a prosthetic mitral valve suitable for transplant during that period meant that most surgeons had to intentionally convert the more "unmanageable" mitral stenosis into mitral regurgitation, a more manageable condition. Facing the threat of possible death as a result of this, Dr. Starr collaborated with Lowell Edwards, a retired engineer, to create a new mechanical valve for patients suffering from mitral stenosis. The pair eventually developed and marketed a simple mechanical device that could be well tolerated by patients suffering from the condition. The device soon gained popularity and many patients who used it could live for more than 30 years after having a valve replacement.

Dr. Starr's story of innovation proves the value of physician involvement in entrepreneurial innovations. His clinical experience afforded him the important insights necessary to making the device reliable, and intuitive for users. Indeed, a study aimed at investigating the pattern of patent applications for medical devices showed that devices with significant physician design involvement were much more effective and comfortable for patients. The study also found that medical startups founded by physicians were much more productive than those started by non-physicians.

Yet, despite these revelations, only few medical institutions place emphasis on entrepreneurial innovations. Most medical institutions have become outdated in this respect and provide students with little or no relevant education or opportunities to pursue creativity or explore their ingenuity.

Chapter 6

PHYSICIANS AS QUALITY IMPROVEMENT LEADERS

ESSENTIALS OF QUALITY IMPROVEMENT

The traditional role of a physician is limited to the diagnosis and treatment of ailments behind the closed doors of hospital wards and within the confines of a physician-patient relationship. Considering present realities, now more than ever this traditional role must be extended to include more organizational, social, and political context, where the diagnosis and treatment of healthcare system failures themselves is as important as that for individual patients!

There's been growing concern over quality improvement in the last decades as evidence of inefficiencies, inadequacies, and uneven quality emerges. Unless physicians are able to understand and influence this broader context, their ability to improve the overall quality of healthcare in an increasingly complex environment will be limited. The ability to understand and exert meaningful influence can be achieved by participating in the emerging science of Quality Improvement. To more permanently alter the balance of power in our favor as physicians, we must be willing to establish strong and visionary leadership in healthcare quality improvement.

While physicians are key to quality improvement efforts, the task of focusing these activities is quite daunting for many reasons, including but not limited to professional pressures. Though most physicians regard quality improvement as a professional responsibility, their quality improvement efforts are usually limited to the patient in front of them or sometimes to a larger population of patients. They tend to focus more on clinical quality and effectiveness, often neglecting broader dimensions of quality, such as general system-wide efficiency, equity, and patient-responsiveness. To overcome these challenges, physicians themselves and healthcare organizations must employ prudent strategies. To succeed requires a comprehension of the relationships between the different quality challenges that plague our healthcare system, the different kinds of errors that lead to them, and how responsive these various kinds of errors may be to different interventions efforts.

There is definitely no shortage of evidence describing the deficiencies in our current healthcare systems. In the US alone, one out of every ten patients admitted to hospitals experiences iatrogenic harm. There are wide variations in quality of care across the country, and some health inequalities are getting worse rather than better. Care is often poorly coordinated and patients don't always experience the level of attention that doctors would regard as acceptable for themselves or their families. Ultimately, resources are wasted, and parts of the workforce demoralized.

Chapter 7

PHYSICIANS AS MANAGERS

OVERVIEW

The healthcare landscape is changing, and so is what is expected from participants. Physicians are expected to deliver top-notch clinical care alongside being able to manage service delivery, oversee budgets, and pushing for quality improvement. Unlike before, this array of expectations is no more merely a choice for physicians who choose to be interested in this topic, but rather an accepted requirement for all physicians.

As we've reiterated throughout this book, a core objective is to prepare physicians for leadership positions within healthcare systems. An important precursor to all-round effective leadership is having good managerial skills. It's therefore imperative that physicians prepare themselves for assuming managerial roles in their organizations well beyond their clinical practice. To ultimately become effective leaders in healthcare, physicians need to possess effective management skills.

We need to understand exactly *why* our participation in management is essential, and the benefits it brings, to our organizations and our patients. Physicians need to understand why being "management suitable" is a necessary evil rather than an irrelevant adventure. Physicians need to understand how the managerial actions taken with or without their participation can negatively or positively impact their professional and personal lives. While "division of labor" and "comparative advantage" in its strictest form made sense in healthcare few years ago, the effectiveness of such a model is questionable in today's world.

So, as physicians, we shouldn't be afraid to mix managerial skills with clinical expertise in order to amass benefits to ourselves, our organizations, and our patient population. Indeed, if we lack these skills, there's a risk that our clinical objectives as physicians may never be met. It's safe to say that management in today's healthcare landscape is far too important to ignore. Also, the approach of "I'm too busy to deal with management" is fast losing touch with present realities. As physicians, we have an obligation to be conscious of the rudiments of effective management and working cohesively in multidisciplinary teams. We must be able to use a variety of resources to play an active role in developing and setting priorities, as well as take the lead in improving healthcare outcomes within our practice.

In recent years, countless strategies have been put forward in an attempt to stimulate physicians' involvement in management. And to some appreciable extent, management topics are gradually being included in undergraduate curricula. Upcoming physicians are indeed becoming more exposed to management knowledge.

Physicians are, more than ever, expected to assume roles related to the management of human as well as financial resources in healthcare organizations, especially in hospitals. Surely, alternating between their management responsibilities and clinical practice (including their roles as physician-teachers and physician-researchers) can lead to conflicting roles. Nonetheless, their presence and active participation in healthcare management is crucial to shaping the future healthcare system. Physicians bring important skills and values such as ethical judgment, observation, analysis, and problem-solving into management positions.

Physicians now provide more than just therapeutic care for patients but also expert opinion for other physicians and health care providers. Historically, physicians have always had a leadership role within healthcare. However, in recent years there's been a significant increase in the number of physicians assuming major managerial responsibilities. Physicians across different specialties now advise governments at different levels on policies related to healthcare, including but not limited to medical practice, effectiveness and efficiency of medical care, appropriateness of care, and organization of the healthcare system.

But the greatest increase in physicians' involvement in managerial activities is taking place in hospitals. Different stakeholders within hospital settings are recognizing the advantages of physician participation in management and the need to work together to make appropriate managerial decisions, with the interests of patients at the forefront. As a matter of fact, the traditional "dual hierarchy" paradigm with medical staff forming a second line of authority after the administrative staff, is fast becoming ineffective and obsolete.

We're in the middle of a paradigm shift, and to some extent, we've experienced one already. There's a trend that's fast becoming the new "way of being." Different hospitals are now experimenting various ways to integrate physicians into administrative decision-making. Physicians now routinely (and rightly!) participate in issues affecting the entire hospital's strategic planning, operational planning, and quality improvement. Physicians are also now being asked to take up roles as salaried line managers, with positions as vice-president or chief of a department in prospect.

They're also being asked to manage decentralized clinical programs. The trend of appointing more physicians as managers is not only prevalent in the United States, but also in Canada and several other countries. The "new way of things" decision making is decentralized to clinical programs or strategic business units reaffirms the need for physicians' participation in managerial responsibilities. As physicians we must be grounded in this new trend of integrating administrative and clinical decision making, and recognize it as an opportunity to bring clinical expertise to bear in managerial issues.

To cope in our evolving environment, physicians must develop knowledge and skills in policy and political processes when it comes to healthcare. But we must also be grounded in management of finances, management of human resources, organizational design, and systems and program quality improvement. Finally, as physicians, it's important for us to understand the structural framework of health service within which to apply our new management skills, both locally and nationally.

PROBLEMS WITH PHYSICIANS MANAGEMENT SKILLS

The Merriam Webster defines Management as the "act or skill of controlling or making decisions about a business, department, etc." or the people responsible for making those decisions. Though management as an act or skill has been traditionally ascribed to businesses, as we've seen earlier in this book, management is just as important in healthcare settings. Here, management is usually undertaken either as patient management, people management, organizational management or any combination of these. However, irrespective of the category physician managers may find themselves in, they inevitably lack the required skill to carry out their managerial responsibilities effectively.

Throughout their careers, physicians are very much likely to be thrust into complex management and leadership scenarios that their regular academic curricula did not prepare them for. More and more is expected from physicians, but they still lack the necessary skills to navigate real-world situations. The current medical curriculum is still rather delayed in reflecting the rapid changes in healthcare, and adapting to teach vital management and leadership skills.

Whether it's the newly qualified doctor trying to juggle four patients in the emergency room or a physician team leader trying to liaise with team members to achieve a goal, these physicians may not have had sufficient prior training to cope. Whilst most physicians may possess the skills to navigate the most intricate of *clinical* scenarios, their lack of management training is nevertheless a problem.

The current medical curriculum introduces skills that student physicians predict will be invaluable to their future medical careers. But with the responsibilities of physicians continuously evolving, it's becoming more important to take charge and learn to manage a host of complex and unpredictable situations. In the past there was emphasis on the doctor as a transactional leader, yet recent changes in modern medicine increasingly demands that we are *transformational* leaders, empowering peers and seeking to achieve collective organizational change.

There has been an irresistible drive to make patient-centered care an integral part of modern healthcare delivery. As transformational leaders, clinicians must effectively engage both their intra-disciplinary and multi-disciplinary teams. This involves coordinating a variety of professionals and personalities, and understanding team dynamics and motivation to ensure an efficient and positive outcome for both the team and patient.

PHYSICIANS AS STRATEGIC MANAGERS

The dynamics of today's healthcare organizations are fraught with complexities. There's increasing difficulty in satisfying a more progressive, more "aware" and more demanding population, and the need to modify the working dynamics of their organizations to keep pace with the very rapid changes taking place in healthcare.

In the opinion of many physicians, strategic management is a bureaucratic and MBA-worthy undertaking that can only be run from a hospital administrator's office. Their image of strategic management might involve a flurry of unwanted interviews, maybe some retreats, and a few lofty commitments. However, strategic management more properly involves some of the most vital deliberations and decisions that occur in a hospital, or indeed any healthcare organization. Physicians who don't participate in strategic management may find themselves isolated from deliberations and decisions that have direct impacts on them, their patients, and their entire clinical practice. Strategic management is ultimately a leadership tool. For physician leaders, strategic management is not optional, but an indispensable tool that must be mastered.

Physician participation in strategic management can help healthcare organizations adjust to the constraints of a lean economy, rapidly evolving technologies, and a greater than ever need to provide quality services at reasonable prices. Our participation provides a structure for assessing current paradigms and developing a smart approach to boosting revenue while minimizing costs.
It's fast becoming apparent that hospitals and healthcare organizations that have failed to integrate physicians into managerial roles will pay for their inattention in time. In today's world of value-based

demand, integrating physicians into management has never been more crucial.

The future of most healthcare organizations will depend on the ability of physicians and other medical care providers to deliver more effective care in measurable ways. It will also depend on the delivery of more reliable outcomes at lower costs. Physicians, perhaps more than any group, are in an excellent position to develop strategies to deliver that value. Physicians are uniquely positioned, due to their insider knowledge and clinical experience, to understand the trajectory of healthcare markets, and provide insights into how to respond to challenges.

When physicians jointly build strategic initiatives with other stakeholders, they help mediate the risk of falling short in a rapidly changing and increasingly challenging market. Since physicians are highly invested in delivering quality care to patients, and since they possess a broad range of insights into how things could be done effectively, engaging them in strategic management is a natural part of building an effective strategy. Furthermore, since physicians will ultimately be at the forefront of implementing those strategies and managerial decisions, they're positioned to best implement them.

One of the most painful things a physician is routinely asked to do is call the insurance company to fight for what they think is best for patients. Finding a moment to call, and dealing with the automated phone service until you can connect with an actual human being, physicians regularly find themselves in the position of having to explain the complexities of what they're trying do, all the while knowing that the person on the other end of the line will make a decision that ultimately benefits his boss. Not the patient. Not the physician. But a stakeholder motivated primarily by profit.

Insurance and pharmaceutical companies thrive on the system like leeches. But it's doctors who have made room for these various stakeholders to continuously expand their influence in healthcare, and they'll continue to do so until doctors realize that it's the lack of their own initiative and leadership that has allowed it. Insurance companies are not really to blame; rather, doctors have painted themselves into a corner. Innovation, leadership, and entrepreneurship are not easy, especially when they've been largely ignored over 10 to 14 years of training. But the sobering truth is that in our reluctance to take charge, we have allowed a perhaps more untenable situation to take root.

"BUSINESS OF MEDICINE" ISSUES ARE NOW FOREFRONT IN THE MINDS OF MOST PHYSICIANS.

The economic pressure to reduce cost while increasing quality are intensifying across practice environments. The complexity of managing patients with chronic disease and the need for collaboration among multiple physicians is becoming the new normal, as is the focus on patient and staff satisfaction. In short, the role of the physician is changing rapidly. Most medical schools in the United States have adapted their curricula to include team-based approaches. However, graduating students still lack the fundamental business and leadership training needed to effect the changes required to simultaneously maximize quality and reduce cost in clinical practice. Regardless of whether future physicians decide to work in a large healthcare system or choose solo practice, they'll need fundamental knowledge and skills in three key business disciplines: leadership, teamwork, and data analytics.

Without major improvements in operational efficiency, our nation will be unable to fund the cost of providing the highest quality medical care to a demographically older and more diverse population. Accomplishing this will involve much more than improving supply chain costs and shortening hospital stays. It will require right sizing the number of hospitals and specialists, reducing time between procedures, and leveraging information technology in powerful new ways. Healthcare is too diverse across geographies and too fragmented in its structure, but reimbursement for this is done exclusively by management consultants or health plan administrators. Physicians will need to own this process to create the effective, organic change that comes from those closest to patient care and is most trusted by fellow doctors. As difficult as it is to change physician behavior, our observation is that when the process is not led by a physician, the results usually fall short of expectations.

DEVELOPING ROBUST MANAGEMENT SKILLS AS A PHYSICIAN

A lot has been written about professionalism in medicine and a physician's position among the top hierarchy of health professionals. Indeed, in their quest to push for improved healthcare outcomes, much is expected from physicians in management roles. There's a general belief among healthcare professionals that healthcare organizations will have an improved chance of successfully tackling the plethora of challenges they face if they're managed by people with substantial clinical experience. There are certainly dozens of high-profile studies that support this belief. However, management skills don't necessarily come intuitively. Honing effective and robust management skills takes time and effort.

Currently, too many physicians in management roles rely on their innate instinct, fine-tuned mostly by experience on the job, when dealing with complex managerial issues and situations. But the complexities of present management roles demand more than just on-the-job experience or gut feeling. Management-suitable physicians with the hunger to provide high quality leadership in healthcare organizations need to get themselves comfortable with the existing body of management evidence and theory, both at the operational and strategic levels.

Until they're properly acquainted with current management thinking, their approach towards management would be based largely on well intentioned, but vague, principles. It's important that physicians learn management systematically from current academic thought in areas such as negotiation, leadership, innovation, strategic development, marketing, and financial management. This would provide them with a robust platform from which to operate.

There are definitely no shortcuts to successful leadership as managers in healthcare organizations. Nonetheless, not all potential physician managers need to study management theory at degree level before being prepared for management. They can still be ready by carefully identifying and selecting developmental opportunities and by making use of the large body of management thinking and evidence currently available. It's safe to say that physicians possess important built-in skills and values harnessed through their involvement in clinical roles. For example, during our medical and residency training, we learn to analyze and fix problems through a meticulous and analytical approach to diagnosis and treatment. These analytical skills and values are quite important to a physician manager's success in their role, but they must broaden the scope of analysis to include more far-reaching variables.

Traditionally, a physician's analysis in a clinical setting focuses almost totally on the interests of the patient. However, a physician manager's analysis-based decisions must be made in a much broader context and must take into account other variables like the interest of an organizational healthcare program, a department as a whole, a hospital or a whole system. To help physicians gain expertise in management, various organizations must design and offer relevant educational programs, ranging from short courses to graduate university programs in health administration.

As governments become increasingly involved in control of healthcare organizations in order to contain costs on their own part, the medical profession will also have to increase its involvement in policy formation and management of the healthcare system at all levels. The reality on the ground means it's no more a question of *whether* physicians should participate in management of healthcare systems but, rather, *how* to foster their participation. As potential managers, plenty of physicians will face challenges in balancing clinical, advocacy, teaching, and research roles discussed in this book, with management roles. To strike a balance, physician managers must increase their knowledge in a number of critical areas.

POLICY AND POLITICAL PROCESSES

Since government and their policies are usually inextricably intertwined with healthcare, physicians must be political aware. They must be familiar with how health policies are formulated and influenced, and subsequently design strategies to effectively influence this process. This usually involves developing effective ways to engage in meaningful dialogue with government at all levels. Physicians must also be familiar with different economic variables and the ways they affect the healthcare system, the available financial options for reimbursing physicians and funding hospitals operations, and the consequences of these options to their clinical practice and the healthcare system as a whole.

MANAGING AND DEVELOPING OTHERS

Effective management requires the ability to plan and develop not just one's own work but also the work of others. Importantly, it also requires delegating and mentoring skills. In essence, this means physician managers must learn to work more collaboratively — a style that isn't particularly nurtured in a command-and-control environment.

BALANCE OF PATIENT-FOCUSED AND PHYSICIAN-FRIENDLY APPROACHES

One of the most important reasons physicians prefer to be managed by other physicians is because of their ability to see and understand both sides. A regular manager may be isolated from the day-to-day clinical realities of a healthcare establishment, and how it impacts both the physicians and patients. On the other hand, physician mangers are perceived to understand the dynamics of what's needed to keep the physician working at optimum conditions while patients are catered for in the best possible way, all without compromising organizational objectives. Physician managers must develop a sixth sense to understand population-based approaches to health care services and their implications for medical practice and service management.

QUALITY IMPROVEMENT

Quality improvement skills are core to a physician manager's ability to execute overall management roles effectively. To develop robust management skills, physician managers must cultivate a culture of quality improvement. They must actively participate in identifying clinical processes that can be improved as well as play an integral part in implementing quality improvement recommendations.

PROGRAM DEFINITION AND MANAGEMENT

As different health care organizations are hard-pressed to reevaluate their mission, they're able to define their program priorities more clearly. Physicians must participate in and sometimes manage all phases of individual programs — planning, budgeting, evaluation, and outcome.

HOW TO ACQUIRE A STRATEGIC PERSPECTIVE

Basically, a perspective is a way or manner of viewing things, and it's important that every business, including healthcare businesses, use multiple perspectives to form a holistic vision for their organization. Seeing things from a strategic perspective is critical to the success of any healthcare organization. In the business of healthcare, the strategic perspective is usually very important as it helps drives efficiency and builds a competitive mindset within an organization. Leaders of healthcare organizations with fast-paced growth and overall efficiency usually ensure that their operational and management strategy is always based on diverse input. By engaging patients, physicians, and other medical service suppliers, a broad perspective is developed. This gives a 360-degree view of the organization and develops a broad commitment to its success. Planning from a strategic perspective means organizations can develop a range of approaches to common healthcare obstacles.

Acquiring a strategic perspective is not necessarily easy. In health organizations, most physicians and other clinical employees are bombarded with essential daily tasks. While navigating the heaps of day-to-day demands, it becomes almost too easy to miss the big picture. Acquiring a strategic perspective means seeing the healthcare organization as a complex machine with different but equally important parts. It requires taking a step back to consider these parts as a whole. The process of acquiring a strategic perspective is not static, however: as the business evolves, so should the strategies.

A strategic perspective is not the same as an operational perspective. Strategic perspective is particularly focused on wider-reaching, broad, and long-lasting issues that concern the effectiveness and survival of medical practice in the long run. An operational perspective, on the other hand, focuses on achieving day-to-day objectives and short-term activities. Strategic plans are usually not rigid as they meet bottlenecks and obstacles requiring the adaptation and adjustment as the plan is implemented. To be of long-term value, a strategic plan must be seen as an ongoing business process. It must evolve or be modified to reflect changing healthcare variables.

Chapter 8

PHYSICIANS AS HR MANAGERS

Human resources management (HRM) is a broad concept, even within the confines of a healthcare ecosystem. Naturally, understanding this concept would be much simpler if we understand the terms "human resources" and "management." Firstly, we all know that people in work organizations come with a range of skills, abilities, talents, and attitudes. It's obvious that the application of these skills is what influences productivity, quality, and profitability. These people, call them employees or workers, are responsible for setting overall strategies and goals, for the design of work systems, delivery of services, monitoring of quality, allocation of financial resources, and marketing of products and services that such an organization may offer. By virtue of the "resourceful services" they provide, these people therefore become "human resources." That being said, it won't be far from the truth if we say that human resources are the people themselves. Human resources, when pertaining to healthcare, can be defined as the various clinical and non-clinical employees within a healthcare organization who are responsible for public and individual health intervention. Human resources management can basically be seen as the defining of roles and responsibilities of these people, and managing them in ways that maximizes an individual's contribution in line with organizational goals.

THE IMPORTANCE OF HUMAN RESOURCES MANAGEMENT IN HEALTHCARE

Behind every successful organization is an organized and cohesive workforce. This is especially true in the healthcare industry, where the quality of human resource management determines the effectiveness of recruitment, training of staff, and implementation of safety measures. An effective human resources management practice in the healthcare sector means that organizations are orderly and effectively managed overall. When healthcare organizations, especially hospitals, are equipped with a high-quality HR management program, the staffs are much better able to provide outstanding services for their patients. Staff training is usually one of the most crucial roles of human resources within a healthcare organization. An effective human resources management team means that medical staff are adequately trained to deliver high efficiency outcomes.

Similarly, human resources helps to clarify roles and responsibilities, and helps staff adhere to these roles. Imagine being hired in a new job in a hospital and never actually knowing exactly what your new position entails. This happens often, unfortunately, and it's usually both embarrassing and frustrating for the employee. Human resources management can help set things straight if this happens. But the presence of an effective human resources management team would also ensure that this doesn't happen in the first place. How employees of a healthcare organization are managed, both individually and in groups, has an invaluable impact on the overall efficiency of such an organization. It's safe to say that HRM plays a vitally important role in quality improvement as well as in preparing healthcare institutions for industry wide healthcare reforms.

HRM is usually primarily concerned with the development of both individual employees and the organization in which they operate. It involves developing and securing the talents of individual employees as well as the implementation of programs and strategies that enhance cooperation and healthy communication between individual employees. One of the aims of HRM is naturally to nurture human resources in an organization in ways that will foster organizational development. But other roles include job analysis and staffing, effective use of the available workforce, measurement and appraisal of the performance of the workforce, design and implementation of reward systems, and the professional development of employees. It's responsible for complex decisions regarding the attraction, selection, training, assessment, and rewarding of workers. HRM is also concerned with overseeing compliance to organizational culture as well as relevant employment and labor laws.

Within a healthcare setting, human resources management are responsible for:
- Development an efficient legal and ethical management system
- Organizational job design and analysis
- Design of mechanisms for recruitment and selection
- Providing and informing medical staffs of healthcare career opportunities

- Allocating employee benefits
- Designing and implementing employee motivation strategies
- Supervising or participating in negotiations with organized labor
- Termination of employees' employment
- Studying and evaluating emerging and future trends in healthcare
- Participating in strategic planning

Human resources is undeniably the backbone of any healthcare institution. A hospital, for example, could easily be defined by the quality of its staff. The job of ensuring staff quality in a hospital would usually partly rest on the HR units of that hospital. Ensuring that healthcare organizations are manned by people with the right skills and qualities is also the responsibility of the HR unit. Unfortunately, human resources management in most cases doesn't get the priority it deserves in an organization. If left unattended, the consequences of neglecting efficient HRM practice would substantially affect the quality of medical services. The process of HRM planning begins immediately after the conceptualization of a business project, making it as important as any other aspect of healthcare management.

Chapter 9

PHYSICIANS AS LEADERS

PHYSICIAN LEADERSHIP SKILLS

Effective leadership in healthcare requires a range of unique skills, both those which come naturally as well as those that must be acquired. It's important for physicians to identify and explore some of these skills if they are to become effective leaders. These skills can be considered either organizational behavior-based skills as well as analytical ones. However, our discussion on this topic will focus more on the organizational behavior-based skills, since they're generally considered the most important for culture-centered leadership strategies.

Physicians lacking organizational behavior-based skills would surely find it challenging to channel the ideas and goals of stakeholders into solving challenging problems that their organization may face. Another reason for focusing on organizational behavior-based skills is that physicians are less likely to acquire them through regular medical education or clinical practice. In contrast, physicians already possess analytical skills and use them in their daily practice for formulating differential diagnoses, evaluating laboratory and test results, and deciding the best treatment for patients. As a matter of fact, apart from the almost indispensable physician-patient relationship, none or very few other interpersonal leadership skills are emphasized to the same extent as analytical skills in medical education and practice. Nonetheless, effective physician leaders cannot do without interpersonal leadership skills in their quest to achieve their goals using culture-centered approaches.

For instance, rather than just analyzing a decision quantitatively (using analytical skills), a leader should endeavor to motivate others (motivation is an interpersonal leadership skill) to identify challenges and drive problem solving, efficiency, knowledge sharing, and commitment to the organization.

ORGANIZATIONAL BEHAVIOR-BASED SKILLS

- Motivation of followers
- Effective communication
- Team building
- Conflict management
- Culture development
- Analytical skills
- Risk analysis
- Quality control
- Financial expertise

ORGANIZATIONAL BEHAVIOR SKILLS

MOTIVATION

Motivation is an invaluable leadership skill in almost every industry, including healthcare. To lead effectively, physicians need to understand the intricacies of proper motivation and how to use them to bring out the most from other physicians or anyone else in the organization. In the confines of HRM strategies, motivation is a key to stimulating worker potential. Different theories on motivation include content-based and process-based theories. The first focuses on motivating others through fulfilling their needs.

A popular content-based theory developed by Abraham Maslow, — Maslow's Hierarchy of Needs — breaks down human need into five basic levels. These are physiological, security, social, self-esteem, and self-actualization. Maslow defined physiological needs as being the most basic of all, i.e. survival. Similarly, the security needs include shelter and stability, social needs include a yearning for interpersonal relationships, affiliation, and belonging, and self-esteem needs include desiring praise, achievement, and recognition. According to Maslow, the highest need is that of self-actualization or put simply, the fulfillment of one's true human potential. Maslow claimed that individuals must fulfill the more basic needs before they can start focusing on the higher ones. That being said, it then becomes apparent that if physician leaders can identify and fulfill the basic needs of people they lead, they can ultimately stimulate or motivate employees to reach their highest potential. Although there's currently no concrete evidence for Maslow's theory, it nonetheless remains one of the most important content-based theories.

A similar theory that builds on Maslow's theory is that of McClelland. In his Socially Acquired Needs Theory, McClelland identifies three basic needs that humans have, which includes the need for achievement, power, and affiliation. He maintains that achievement-motivated individuals derive satisfaction and motivation from pursuing and reaching their goals. Power-motivated individuals see each situation as a chance to take control (over others or over the mechanisms of an organization) while affiliation-motivated individuals are driven by the joy of harmonious social cohesion and group acceptance. Considering McClelland's perspective, physician leaders can motivate others for greater productivity and efficiency by identifying and fulfilling the unique needs of each worker. It's important to note that there's a wealth of scientific evidence which supports McClelland's theory. It's safe to conclude that a physician's motivation skills depend greatly on their ability to identify and address these needs in others.

Although there are a several other needs-based theories, all of them commonly posit that effectively motivating individuals — in our case, healthcare workers — means understanding the essential needs of those we intend to lead. In the same vein, process-based theories such as the popular expectancy theory, focus on the relationship between increased effort, performance, and outcomes. The expectancy theory directly relates motivation to expectancies, instrumentalities, and valances. Here, expectancies is the idea that an increased effort will lead to an improvement in performance. Instrumentalities is the idea that an improved performance will lead to a particular outcome, and valences is the perceived value of a particular outcome. A physician leader can therefore motivate others by ensuring that increased effort actually leads to better performance, that improved performance actually leads to a better outcome, and that such an outcome ultimately remains valuable.

EFFECTIVE COMMUNICATION SKILLS

Another very important skill a physician leader should possess is effective communication skills. Within healthcare, effective communication encompasses the ability of a physician leader to convey feelings, concerns, concepts, ideas, and directions to others in ways they can understand. It's the ability of a physician leader to comprehend and appreciate the perspective, ideas and concerns of others. It has a lot to do with a physician's ability to discern important issues about other healthcare stakeholders and design communication patterns that are beneficial to everyone involved.

To participate in decision-making processes, collaborative activities, or motivational strategies, a physician leader must be able to communicate effectively. An intelligent agenda, goal or aim means nothing if it's not communicated to others in ways they understand and put into operation. The content of an idea alone is not enough. A million-dollar idea or brilliant message may mean absolutely nothing if the people it's intended for don't understand and interpret it in the way it was intended. This is why it's essential for a physician leader to understand their audience and communicate in ways that can be clearly understood.

A physician leader with effective communication skills should not only be able to verbalize thoughts and intentions clearly, but also facilitate communications between themselves and others. They should be able to create an environment that fosters knowledge sharing in their organization, actively sharing information in a thoughtful way, and creating opportunities for the best decisions to be made. Knowledge sharing has been proven to significantly build trust and cooperation among stakeholders, as well as promote the influx of useful new information, ultimately improving performance.

Nonetheless, there are some established cognitive and motivational factors that hinder knowledge sharing. A good example of a cognitive barrier is a difference in expertise level among parties that would otherwise share information. Physician leaders can overcome such barriers by using individuals with intermediate levels of knowledge to mediate and by encourage two-way communication. Apart from cognitive factors, motivational factors like lack of incentives, status hierarchies, and lack of trust can greatly hinder effective communication. Fortunately, physician leaders can overcome motivational barriers by increasing incentives as well as encouraging people to focus more on organizational goals while de-emphasizing status distinctions. As a practical example, deemphasizing status differences between nurses and physicians in hospitals could encourage nurses to share critical knowledge on a patient's condition with physicians, and to question flawed decisions.

TEAM BUILDING

To put it succinctly, team building is the process of creating useful synergy and collaboration between individuals who may have a common goal. It's the ability of a physician leader to organize and nurture a diverse group of people in a way that promotes synergy between individual performance attributes. In healthcare, team spirit helps to facilitate the sharing of useful information and also promotes constructive criticism. Effective physician leaders must recognize the importance of team performance, actively invest in the idea of teamwork, and actively participate in such a team.

A physician leader's ability to build effective teams is critical to achieving organizational goals, since most important decisions would normally require the input of different parties with unique ideas and equally unique perspectives. Physician leaders should be able to play a critical role in team building not only by engaging members towards the team goals, but also by providing an environment that fosters trust, clearly setting the foundation of ideals by which the team will function.

Physician leaders who want to develop the skills to build and participate in effective teams must understand how effective teams actually work. According to Bruce Tuckman's traditional model of team development, teams go through 5 stages of development, namely: forming, storming, norming, performing, and adjourning. The forming phase is characterized by orientation. This is where team members identify opportunities and challenges, and then agree on different goals and how to tackle identified challenges or take on different tasks. The storming phase is characterized by conflict, disagreements, and personality clashes. The norming kicks in after conflicts and personality clashes are resolved, leading to better cohesion between team members. This phase is characterized by harmony as a result of greater intimacy. The performing stage is where team norms and roles are executed and is usually characterized by decision making. Understanding these different stages can help physician leaders steer teams in ways that maintain focus and commitment.

CONFLICT MANAGEMENT

Going by Bruce Tuckman's model of group development, conflicts within a group may be inevitable. A physician leader must consequently possess the skill needed to manage conflicts, whether that's within a team, a larger group, individuals, or an entire organization. There's a wealth of studies showing that conflict is necessary for cultural change, adaptation, and success. Conflicts in a healthcare setting could either be a task conflict (creative tension) or affective (relationship) conflict. Task conflict is a necessary evil and an important part of problem solving that propels decision making and change.

In his book, *Leadership Without Easy Answers*, Heifitz explains that, "Conflict and heterogeneity are resources for social learning. Although people may not come to share one another's values, they may learn vital information that would ordinarily be lost to view without engaging the perspectives of those who challenge them." Task conflict forces individuals with a similar goal to explore all aspects and approaches to solving a problem while ensuring that no unforeseen consequences are ignored. It helps to stimulate optimum performance and enhance problem solving when enough conflict exists to unravel different approaches and perspectives, but not so much that it stifles discussion.

On the other hand, affective or relationship conflict is almost always bad for business. Nothing particularly good usually comes from this type of conflict within a team or an organization. Affective conflict revolves around personal attacks and personality clashes rather than disagreements about the task at hand. It could be entirely irrelevant to organizational goals with no constructive impact. Consequently, a physician leader should be able to identify and resolve any level of affective conflict. Physician leaders develop and nurture conflict resolution strategies that help them manage task conflict while eliminating affective conflict. Physician leaders need the ability to focus on the issues at hand rather than the people discussing the issues, on data and not on opinions, and know how to put the common goals of groups and organizations above individual goals.

However, as counterintuitive as it might sound, excessive cohesion can be just as bad as conflict. When excessively high cohesion causes everyone within a group to agree too easily on complex decisions, then the entire group is likely to have overlooked different perspectives or contradictory but important details. When this happens, it leads to a condition known as "groupthink." This is a condition that arises within individuals, teams or groups wherein their desire for harmony or conformity leads to a rather dysfunctional decision-making outcome. In his 1972 book, *Victims of Groupthink*, Irving Janis, a research psychologist from Yale University, describes groupthink as "a mode of thinking that people engage in when they are deeply involved in a cohesive in-group, when the members' strivings for unanimity overrides their motivation to realistically appraise alternative courses of action."

Abba Eban, a former Israeli Foreign Minister, once said that, "Consensus is what everyone agrees to say collectively... and, no one believes individually." The desire for harmony within a group by a physician leader is normal, but when harmony is oversubscribed, it undermines objective decision making. A physician leader must therefore possess a fundamental understanding of conflicts as well as group harmony and conformity to be able to successfully steer the affairs or groups within an organization, or the entire organization itself.

CULTURE DEVELOPMENT

Though quite subtle, less understood, and far less put into practical use, understanding organizational culture is a foundational prerequisite for understanding and even predicting how things will be within an organization. It gives a physician leader an invaluable insight into existing patterns, trends, values, norms, organizational dynamics, way of life and, to some extent, the mechanisms of operation in an organization. In their book, *Strategic Management*, Hill and Jones described organizational culture as "the specific collection of values and norms that are shared by people and groups in an organization and that control the way they interact with each other and with stakeholders outside the organization." Therefore, a clear understanding of the underlying culture of an organization can be invaluable in predicting or controlling how individuals within that organization respond to different situations, and how they interact with one another.

Apart from understanding the organizational culture, an effective physician leader should be able to mold the culture in ways that are beneficial to organizational goals. They should be able to steer an organization's underlying culture in areas like interpersonal relationships, communication, acceptable attributes, and so on. A strong culture will usually include values such as transparency, trust, and cooperation. Lencioni also explains in his book, *The Five Temptations of a CEO*, that an effective leader must be willing to take the initiative in showing vulnerability. With such actions, a leader portrays vulnerability as an acceptable attribute, thereby setting the stage for the development and nurturing of trust. Lencioni stated in his book that leaders must "know that the best way to get results is to put their weaknesses on the table and invite people to help them minimize those weaknesses."

Nurturing this type of organizational culture is quite important for patient care. A silent but dangerous problem that plagues clinical practice is the fact that physicians and other healthcare providers fear admitting their mistakes. Exacerbated by a dangerous litigation culture within healthcare, this fear prevents healthcare professionals from admitting and subsequently analyzing mistakes and making improvements. The fear of legal repercussions encourages medical professionals to hide mistakes rather than identifying and working to reduce or ameliorate them. All in all, it's vital for physician leaders to understand the cultural values within the healthcare systems that they operate in, and use this understanding in ways that will most benefit patients and those being led. Developing and nurturing a strong organizational culture can help a physician leader to positively direct the actions of those he leads, and help identify specific areas in need of improvement, either by an individual or the organization at large.

ANALYTICAL SKILLS

Despite the emphasis we've placed on explaining organizational behavior-based skills, this doesn't undermine the importance of decision-based analytical skills. It's true that physicians acquire a wealth of analytical skills throughout their education, and many physicians consider analytical skills as being intuitive, at least to them. However, the context of analytical thinking is drastically changed as a physician becomes an organizational leader. It immediately digresses from just evaluating therapeutic care and possible clinical outcomes, and shifts towards evaluating possible outcomes of decisions, weighing their alternatives, analyzing risks, and allocating resources in ways that are efficient and beneficial to patients care.

Lots of analytical skills are taught during a physician's regular education, but leadership-worthy analytical skill are in most cases absent. This is problematic as this type of skill is fundamental to leadership in general. Without analytical skills, a leader in healthcare or any field is likely to fail in making educated decisions about crucial policy changes, investments, or restructuring. In most situations, tasks requiring these skills are outsourced or relegated to accountants, consultants or engineers. Considering this, leaders erroneously assume that mastery in analytical skills isn't particularly necessary. But physician leaders must in fact possess a reasonable level of these skills to analyze, interpret, and share information so they can take the best course of action. Though the context is somewhat different, physician leaders can still apply analytical skills gained from regular medical education and practice to address not only patient diagnosis and treatment, but also analyze decisions. Below is a brief outline of the important analytical skills a physician leader should develop: quality control, risk management, and financial expertise.

QUALITY CONTROL

Quality loss and system failure stem mostly from poor quality control and a poor risk management framework. Quality control is concerned with the methods of identifying areas experiencing quality lost, to quantify that loss, and to make conscious efforts to reduce it. Here, a good organizational culture, as earlier discussed, comes into play. A good example of this outside of healthcare is the Toyota Production System's Kaizen concept. The Kaizen concept is all about frequent improvement by identifying and fixing faults and inefficiencies. Also, as we discussed in organizational culture, covering up problems only leads to additional costs. Inefficiencies and errors should rather be seen as opportunities for improvement.

Quality control is just as applicable to patient care as it is to Toyota's assembly line.

RISK MANAGEMENT

Closely related to quality control is risk management. It involves the evaluation of the possibility and mechanisms of system failures, the quantification of the possible impact of such failures, and the determination of the most effective ways to ameliorate the severity or else totally eliminate the likelihood of such a failure. While little errors in Toyota's assembly line could cause a popping trunk, similar "little" errors in clinical care could unfortunately be fatal. Things like injuries to patients during surgery is a very basic example of "system failure" which needs to be foreseen. The impact of this failure could range from serious injury to death, including all associated costs, both emotional and financial. Considering the devastating implications of medical errors on both patients' well-being and overall healthcare cost, coupled with America's hostile litigation culture, risk management skills are definitely an invaluable tool in a physician leader's war chest.

FINANCIAL EXPERTISE

As a business, financial expertise is just as important in healthcare as it is on Wall Street. Being put in positions of decision making, physician leaders must understand the financial implications of decisions they make or participate in. Doing so requires a reasonable understanding, if not expertise, of things like interest rates, financial statements, billing, taxes, budgets, and profit margins. This understanding is necessary for physician leaders who might need to communicate with financial experts within healthcare systems. It's also important when dealing with administrators or managers whose main concern is the bottom line. Financial expertise helps during project negotiations because stakeholders are more likely to agree if the financial realities of a project can be adequately portrayed, especially in ways that are beneficial to stakeholders and other decision makers. That being said, physicians must come to terms with the fact that to lead effectively, they must understand and speak the language of finance. As an example, to add another care-provider/physician/nurse-practitioner in a particular outpatient service line, the doctor needs to devise a business plan that acknowledges the financial implications for the department/organization, improve access time for patients, enhances customer care and possibly addresses employee satisfaction and physician retention in the organization. Getting things done becomes so much easier if the physician leader understands what the chief financial officer or the chief executive officer considers before approving the new requested position.

A more wide-reaching example concerns reimbursement packages for various specialties. This is considered a major setback for many doctors and their lack of enthusiasm means limited expansion in these specialties. Approaching this problem from a financial perspective may turn things around. For example, a medicine hospitalist service proposes to provide not only the major Internal Medicine admission service but also offers to become the primary service for various specialties like orthopedics, ID, and gastroenterology, so that all the general medical management would be handle by the hospitalists with the specialty service providing the specialized recommendations as needed.

A business plan could be generated with strategic analysis for length of stay, readmission rate, infection rate, mortality, and long-term morbidity as outcome measures. After the initiative, the largest and most financially viable service for a hospital could be identified. The hospitalist service can work with the CFO to get more APP coverage, better FTE support, improved financial packages, and coverage schedules in return for the high-value care being provided. Financial data and good strategic analysis are critical to these negotiations. With proper financial skill, physicians can convert adversity into opportunity.

Chapter 10

TRANSFORMING DOCTORS INTO LEADERS

For a lot of physicians, the position of a formal leader within a healthcare community or organization may not be a desired role. However, the truth remains that all physicians are leaders, regardless of whether they're in salaried or private practice, the size of their private practice, and whether or not to show interest in the larger healthcare economy. Astute physicians meticulously and objectively analyze their own strengths and flaws to better optimize their role in each patient's care plan. Through a similar evaluation process, physicians can establish a fitting role for themselves within the broader healthcare system.

As noted earlier, many practicing physicians don't gain on-the-job experience of traditional leadership. Due to the rapidly increasing demand for physician leaders, they often get directly promoted into leadership roles to either manage others or oversee a business unit in a healthcare organization. This means they skip levels and stages in the leadership pipeline, thereby losing out on the experience and expertise needed to execute the responsibilities of their new roles. They find themselves in a new role that requires skills they simply haven't developed.

Their newfound roles usually require the ability to plan their own work and the work of others, while being able to delegate effectively and make time to coach others. It also requires taking on "healthcare business leadership" which includes understanding business operations, financials, and so on. Succeeding in this new healthcare business leadership role demands a more collaborative way of doing things and the ability to take an enterprise view, effectively balancing short- and long-term concerns. The military styled "command and control" environment that physicians grow up and operate in does not particularly foster these skills. Also, the transition to management and leadership could be especially challenging for physician leaders who continue to deliver clinical care.

This usually eats up the time they would have used to plan, delegate, and execute other leadership responsibilities. Understandably, most physicians would end up prioritizing the clinical care part of their jobs, paying less attention to the part of their jobs that involve leading others. This usually results in micromanagement challenges, knee-jerk decision making, and high turnover due to a lack of feedback or support of their direct reports. It's now common for physician leaders to say, "I just don't have time for that" when asked how much time they put into planning, delegating, and directing the work of others, and to mentor and give feedback.

There are various ways to transform physicians into individuals capable of leading, managing, and developing others. Some of them include specific skill building through training, using an executive coach, providing developmental feedback and investing in the difficult and important work of clarifying the responsibilities and roles of every member of the team. Fortunately, a lot of these skills can be learnt in workshops, and online coaching sessions or educational forums, whether virtual or in-person.

In terms of executive coaching, high potential physician leaders are usually identified and given special continuous coaching by an executive coach. The work of the executive coach is to help them gain self-awareness, set clear goals, reach their development targets, unlock their potentials and act as a sounding board. There's a wealth of evidence showing that executive coaching can be quite effective in developing physician leaders, especially when it's provided at the right time. It's effective because it usually focuses on the specific needs of the physician leader, using a learning style suitable for them, usually delivered at times that work with their schedule. Because this coaching is administered while leaders are still actively participating in leadership roles, it's easier for them to adapt acquired knowledge on the go and use it in tackling specific situations in real time.

However, this type of approach to leadership development involves significant investment and can be counterproductive if certain factors are not considered. To be specific, there are a few factors that have the potential to derail the success of executive coaching:

WHEN THE LEADER ISN'T READY

Sometimes, hospitals or healthcare organizations may try to transform high potential physicians into effective leaders by throwing them into an executive coaching process. When leadership coaching is pushed on a physician leader who isn't ready or doesn't want it, the odds of success decline drastically. Forced development has an almost nonexistent chance of success. Unless healthcare organizations can be candid and compassionate with their physician leaders about issues and possibilities, throwing a coach their way will almost never yield good results. Like the saying goes, "When the student is ready, the teacher will appear."

WHEN THE LEADER HAS NO TIME TO PAUSE

A physician's schedule is usually choked up and physicians are quite busy by default. An additional layer of professional obligations, like taking part in leadership coaching, can be overkill on a physician's schedule. Coupled with the fact that physicians are required to maintain a high degree of clinical excellence and eminence, this extra work load could increase the risk of them burning out. Successful leadership coaching cannot be squeezed into a calendar with no free spaces.

THE DYAD MODEL

Similarly, in the quest to transform physicians into effective leaders, some healthcare organizations have adopted a model known as "dyad." Unlike executive coaching, a physician and a nonclinical business leader share leadership of a business unit or an entire domain within a healthcare organization. The dyad model usually involves pairing clinical and administrative leaders, whereby both serve as co-leaders or with one reporting to the other, to run a market or a business unit. Under this model, some healthcare organizations use a form of dual management structure, one aimed at overseeing the clinical domain and the other at overseeing the business domain.

The aim of the dyad model is to ensure that healthcare organizations have the presence of both clinical expertise and business expertise in their leadership ranks. However, in the search for an effective way to transform physicians into effective leaders, the dyad model is not the optimal solution. While it's worked surprisingly well for a number of organizations, it could cause some delinquency, ultimately raising a number of challenges. This model is usually criticized because it gives room for physician leaders to abscond from learning about the business of healthcare. This means that with the dyad model a physician can avoid learning critical financial, operational, and management skills, limiting their future leadership potential. One of the foundational ideas of the dyad model is to get the physician, who is the clinical leader, to learn from the administrative leader through constant interaction, cooperation, and friendly oversight. However, several challenges plague this model, including power struggles, differences in priorities, and in some cases dramatically conflicting messages to the units of the organization they lead.

To successfully employ the dyad model, there need to be role clarity as well effective communication and collaboration skills, i.e. skills that physicians do not usually have. My perspective on the issue is that doctors need to have a vision and a 5 to 10 year plan that aligns with the organizational goals on how they want the unit or program to run. Often, a visionary can work with administrators by diplomatically learning the skills and driving the ship, while strengthening partnership with their dyad.

Considering the flaws of the above model; it's obvious that it would be more economically sustainable for a healthcare organization to have a single effective physician overseeing (or leading) both the clinical and administrative responsibilities of that organization. If this isn't feasible, an administrator can be added as a partner, but with role clarity. It then becomes important for healthcare organizations to build an adequate pipeline of physicians to gradually but steadily transition into effective leaders.

To build such a pipeline, a healthcare organization's talent management strategy must provide a favorable transitional career path for younger physicians with leadership potential or those with such aspirations. Currently, these opportunities have been rather opportunistic but could definitely be more effective if they're consciously targeted and more intentional.

For example, Kaiser Permanente, now a considerably huge group of hospitals in the U.S., was struggling during the late 1990s. According to reports from the organization, its financial performance and clinical outcomes were rapidly declining. Many celebrated and topnotch physicians started exiting. Things kept going from bad to worse until a new medical director revamped the organization's physician leadership development programs. The revamping process involved identifying potential leaders and putting them through a carefully structured pipeline. In about five years, several impeccable leaders were already developed, immediately improving clinical outcomes. Consequently, the organization blossomed with increased patient satisfaction, lower staff turnover, and improved financial performance especially evidenced in the increase of its annual net profit rising from zero to $87 million.

Chapter 11

FUTURE PROSPECTS

The industry-wide demand for physician leaders is at a critical level. However, even in the face of increasing demand, the healthcare ecosystem is unfortunately showing inadequacies in its attention towards physician leadership. The level of investment needed to transform physicians into leaders (as well as maintain their supply) has been generally abysmal. Building an effective and reliable pipeline of physician leaders at all levels requires enormous investment in time, resources, and attention. Healthcare organizations and relevant stakeholders need to start making this investment now, if they want a continuous stream of leadership-worthy physicians who can run key organizational business units with great skills.

Failure to make this investment means healthcare organizations risk seeing key leadership roles fall into the hands of executives who aren't knowledgeable enough for the job. Healthcare organizations must focus on building leadership capacity, management skills and strategic perspectives in physicians with leadership potential or leadership aspirations. Clinical organizations that do so will be, perhaps more than ever, ready to face the realities of the current and future healthcare landscape.

Medical leadership by physicians is becoming more common and also more important. A report by the American College of Physician Executives indicates that a little above five percent of hospital Chief Executive Officers are now physicians, with that number rapidly increasing under the value-based system. To indicate its importance, the Medical schools at Duke University, the University of Kentucky, Harvard University, Cornell, and the University of Wisconsin pay much attention to medical leadership, currently offering courses like marketing, accounting, and management training alongside regular clinical coursework.

Leadership of medical institutions are also becoming increasingly important partly because physicians relate best to other physicians. Consequently, physicians who can acquire some expertise in the administrative aspects of healthcare are invaluable to the healthcare system because they can use their dual expertise to overcome one of its most lingering challenges – bridging the unhealthy gap that exist between administrators and physicians.

Many physicians are natural problem solvers, so moving into leadership roles with problems to solve is something they might find quite appealing. However, as we already know, the transition from clinical care to leadership isn't always easy. It's important to note our choice of words, the word "leader" rather than "manager" is used. Those may be similar, especially in the context of this book, but they're two different terms. A leader must possess the ability to affect change in a positive manner.

A leader has the ability to affect change in a positive manner. A leader inspires those around them and encourages a willingness to improve. A leader has goals, drive, and commitment - and the skills to achieve them. A manager oversees the day-to-day operations of an organization. Yes, good managers are important, but we desperately need good leaders.

In summary, the healthcare system will flourish if there are partnerships and collaborations among various experts ranging from dynamic managers, innovators, programmers, engineers, coders, billers, caregivers, nurses, providers, physicians, and more. With artificial intelligence knocking on the door, the demand is greater than ever for physician leaders who are visionaries able to lead the transition of the current archaic healthcare system into a high-value, outcomes based, customer-centric, efficient, and innovative future.

CONCLUSION

For efficient healthcare delivery and medical care to keep up with the pace of the healthcare economy, physicians also need to train themselves in areas outside of medicine. As we've seen in the different perspectives portrayed in this book, all physicians are leaders, to some degree. They may lack some of the qualities of effective leaders, but they possess the capacity to become productive leaders. As a matter of fact, physicians possess the intellect, discipline, and ethical background to become quality leaders. However, because leadership skills are not particularly emphasized during their training and practice, doctors approach most problems and situations with a technical solution in mind. However, most challenges within a healthcare setting require adaptive leadership. This type of leadership is necessary to guide healthcare staff and organization cultures through problems and towards solutions to which an easy technical solution may not exist.

The modern physician must be able to research, teach, manage, advocate, and ultimately lead. Leadership is a multi-paradigm concept. Physician leaders should possess the skills to teach and to empower others to confront the challenges they face, at least within the confines of a medical ecosystem, if not beyond. These skills are usually not innate, but they can be acquired through conscious and targeted learning. Physician leaders must possess the analytical abilities to negotiate more than just daily clinical care. If physicians are to exert valuable influence on any realm of healthcare development in the future, effective physician leaders who possess and understand these skills must emerge.

The responsibilities therefore fall on medical education organizations, healthcare organizations, and in my humble opinion, on physicians themselves to take necessary steps to cultivate these invaluable skills. Knowing the value of leadership, the impact it can have on yours and life of others, will change the mindset among clinicians. This book was just a small effort in changing that mindset.

Recognizing the importance of these leadership skills is a necessary first step towards undertaking this responsibility. Participation in conferences, coaching seminars, online courses, and reading books is usually the avenue for physicians to engage with these skills. Some healthcare organizations even provide courses and certification on physician leadership. Unfortunately, the reality remains that these types of courses alone are not nearly enough. Systematic training and continuous application of these skills is necessary to develop and nurture competent physician leaders. It will have to start with doctors willing to get involved in other arenas of healthcare, outside of the domains of patient-physician encounters and operations theaters.

Doctors will have to understand *why* their involvement in leadership is critical, not only for their own career, personal growth, and self-worth, but also to navigate the healthcare system out of its current crisis.

Healthcare organizations can also help foster strong physician leadership skills by exposing physician to all aspects of decision making, management, and leadership. Many healthcare and medical institutions have already modeled their internal leadership structures and programs to help achieve such leadership objectives, and such models can certainly be replicated en masse across the country. The Mayo and Cleveland Clinic models are solid examples of physician leadership being at the core of how these hospital systems function. A recent publication from the University of Texas, Austin confirmed that hospitals listed on U.S. News World reports that were led by physician executives had higher quality ratings and bed-usage performance compared to hospitals led by non-physician leaders, while there was no difference on revenue numbers.

Physicians must be proactive in helping themselves and their organizations to learn about the best ways to lead. Similarly, medical schools and residency programs must place priority on the development of physician leaders by incorporating leadership skills into the curriculum. Fortunately, this is beginning to happen at certain medical institutions, and these programs must be expanded and replicated in other institutions. This ensures that those who are motivated to pursue leadership can cultivate the necessary skills right during their medical training. More of such programs across the country will give the physician leaders of tomorrow a strong background in both clinical and managerial expertise, so they're able to better shape policies in healthcare delivery.

However, the main reason for publishing this book is to introduce various concepts and perspectives for the future breed of hard-working physician. Mainly, to make them aware of what's out there in the "real world" and how can they flourish in that environment. Another reason I wanted to share my perspective was to make newly graduating doctors aware that being a great physician is just one aspect of what will be required of you, and how successful you'll be. The other aspects, which you were not trained in the many years of studying and training, are hopefully shared in this book.

As doctors, we need to realize that the fields of administrative and management sciences, sales and marketing, software programming, artificial intelligence, accounts and finances, and entrepreneurship are just as scientific and evidence based as the field of medicine, and learning these other skills will transform how we look at our roles within the medical profession and in society in general. Without leadership, doctors may ultimately become mere caregivers and technical consultants in the healthcare ecosystem. We have already seen the implications of this; it's high time for us as a doctor community to evolve with changing times.

www.ingramcontent.com/pod-product-compliance
Lightning Source LLC
LaVergne TN
LVHW041545070426
835507LV00011B/933